BUD'S SECRET GARDEN RETREAT

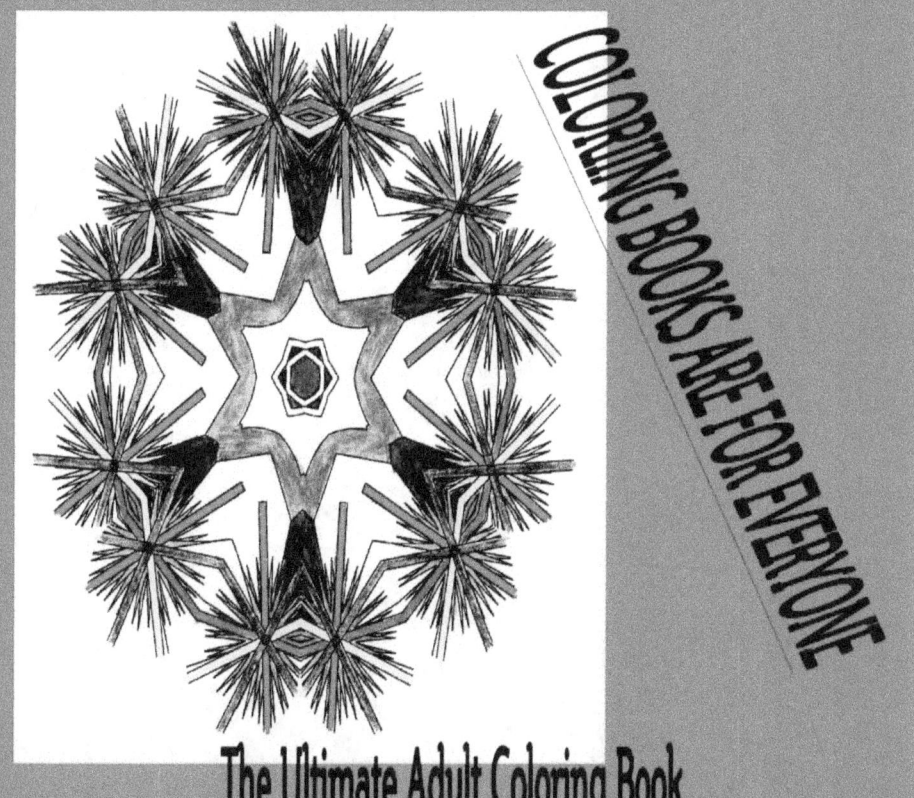

COLORING BOOKS ARE FOR EVERYONE

The Ultimate Adult Coloring Book

Charles L. (Bud) Evans

BUD'S SECRET GARDEN RETREAT

CHARLES L.(BUD) EVANS

INTRODUCTION

Hi, I am Bud Evans and old Montana redneck. There will be a few things different about this coloring book, but the big one is that I will allow you to photocopy pages for your own families use. I I really don't think that this is important thing to put in the introduction, but it's really meaningless. Because you would copy them anyway so I just as well give you permission. You have my permission as the author of this color book to copy any of the pages for your family use.

I am doing this color book to make some money. There is a real use for adult coloring books as they can be a therapeutic agent to a busy mind and a full schedule. Now I thought I'd just throw one of these things together do the work and get paid for it. I discovered in the process of creating these images that I really enjoyed the work. I plan to create at least 10 of these coloring books by the end of September.

You will find a link at the end of the Kindle edition book to the PDF file for these images.

The best way to purchase this book is through Amazon as a paperback.

I have a little story to tell you. One of my daughters was working on her Master's degree and working full-time, was told this. When she was studying she could take a break every half hour and a good thing to do would be to relax and color something. That sound like a really good idea to me.

Now personally I am not a very good colorer. My seven-year-old grandson does a much better job coloring than I do. I have decided to do it for one reason, it relaxes me.

There is no right way or wrong way to color. Just do what you enjoy. Don't be too much of a perfectionist. You can use colored pencils, crayons, markers and some people even use charcoal. Whatever you want is okay. Some days you just want to do it differently.

Again the link for the PDF for the ebook edition is in the end of the book. Please read the section on legal disclaimers and the rest of the legal garbage.

Copyright Notice

All contents of **Benton City Consulting LLC** website or written materials are protected by intellectual property law, including international copyright and trademark laws.

We do not grant rights to any article, book, eBook, document, blog post, software, application, art, graphics, images, video, webinar, recording or other materials viewed or listened to through or from **Benton City Consulting LLC.** If you post to our blog, you surrender all rights to the content once it appears on **Benton City Consulting LLC** website.

YOU MAY NOT MODIFY, COPY, REPRODUCE OR DISTRIBUTE THE MATERIAL ON OUR WEBSITE. You may not sell or modify the material or reproduce, distribute, or otherwise use the material in any way. You are granted a nonexclusive, nontransferable, revocable license to use **Benton City Consulting LLC** materials only for private, personal, noncommercial reasons. You may print or download material for your own non-commercial use. Moreover, you agree not to modify or delete any copyright or proprietary notices from the materials you print or download from **Benton City Consulting LLC**

As a user at **Benton City Consulting LLC** website and of other informational material, you agree to use any products and services offered in a manner consistent with all applicable local, state and Federal laws and regulations. Our website prohibits conduct that might constitute a criminal offense, give rise to civil liability or otherwise violate any law.

Unless allowed by a written agreement, you may not post or transmit advertising or commercial solicitation on our website.

COPYRIGHT WARNING: The legal notices and administrative pages on this website, including this one, have been drafted by the Law Offices of Douglas Slain in October, 2012. **[Benton City Consulting LLC** has paid to license the use of these legal notices and administrative pages for your protection and ours. This material may not be used in any way for any reason; unauthorized use is policed via Copyscape to detect violators.

QUESTIONS/COMMENTS/CONCERNS: If you have any questions about the contents of this page, or simply wish to reach us for any other reason, you may do so by using our Contact information.

Benton City Consulting LLC

108 Acord Road, Benton City, Wa, 99320

budpersonal@gmail.com

Disclaimer

Privacy and Confidentiality

We will take all reasonable precautions to protect the confidentiality of visitor's personal information. We will not use or disclose personal information without users' consent unless authorized by law, and we will not sell, rent, or share personal information about users of our site. Please consult our privacy policy for further information and details.

Our privacy policy clearly describes when and how we collect personal information on the site, the purposes for which we collect this information, with which it will be shared, and how the information will be used.

Personal Information

As used in this Disclaimer, the term "personal information" means any information we collect that can be linked to the user as an individual. That includes mailing address, e-mail account, Internet IP address, demographic information, any unique numerical identifier, and personal information.

We take commercially reasonable precautions to protect the confidentiality of user's personal information. We do not disclose personal information without user's consent unless authorized by law, and we will not sell, rent, or share user's personal information.

This website may track visitor viewing habits to gauge popularity of content and identify trends.

Google Adsense and the DoubleClick DART Cookie

Google, as a third party advertisement vendor, may use cookies to serve ads on **any Benton City Consulting LLC WEBSITE**. The use of DART cookies by Google enables them to serve adverts to visitors that are based on their visits to this website as well as other websites on the internet.

To opt out of the DART cookies you may visit the Google ad and content network privacy policy at the following URL http://www.google.com/privacy_ads.html tracking of users through the DART cookie mechanisms are subject to Google's own privacy policies.

Email

We give clear instructions for subscribing and unsubscribing to e-mail alerts and e-newsletters.

Please see out Anti-spam policy for more information.

Third Parties

We will clearly disclose any significant business relationships between **any Benton City Consulting LLC** and partnering organizations.

Unless stated, you should assume that we at **Benton City Consulting LLC** are not affiliated with any company, person, or organization of any kind mentioned on this **any Benton City Consulting LLC WEBSITE** in any way.

All names of people, trademarks, service marks, company names and brand names are property of their respective owners and are used in editorial commentary as permitted by U.S. law.

Web Links

This Website may contain hypertext links to other websites and information created and maintained by others. These links are only provided for your convenience. **Benton City Consulting LLC** does not control or guarantee the accuracy, completeness, relevance, or timeliness of any information or privacy policies posted on these linked websites.

In addition, hyperlinks to particular items do not reflect their importance, and are not an endorsement of the other individuals or organizations sponsoring the websites, the views expressed on the websites, or the products or services offered on the websites

Benton City Consulting LLC reviews this Website periodically for broken or out-of-date links. Any and all links may be posted, altered, or removed at any time. To report problems with links on the website, or for more information about this policy, please contact us at the address listed at the end of this notice.

Earnings and Income Statements

Benton City Consulting LLC has made no promises, suggestions, projections, representations or guarantees whatsoever about future prospects or earnings that readers of **any Benton City Consulting LLC WEBSITE** may garner as a result of visiting this website, nor has **Benton City Consulting LLC** authorized any such projection or representation by anyone else.

Any earnings or income statements, or any earnings or income examples, are only estimates of what our authors and/or contributors thinks you, the reader, may earn. There is no assurance you will do as well as stated in any examples. You must accept the entire risk of not doing as well as the information provided. This applies whether the earnings or income examples are monetary in nature or pertain to advertising credits which may be earned.

There is no assurance that any prior successes or past results as to earnings or income will apply, nor can any prior success be used as an indication of your future success or results from any of the information, content, or strategies. Any and all claims or representations as to income or earning are not to be considered as "average earnings."

You understand that this website has not been available for purchase long enough to provide an accurate earnings history.

Your Success or Lack of Same

Your success in using the information or strategies provided by this website depends on a variety of factors. **any Benton City Consulting LLC WEBSITE** does not guarantee or imply that you will have any earnings at all.

Internet businesses involve unknown risks. You may not rely on any information presented on this website unless you do so with the knowledge and understanding that you can experience significant losses.

Forward Looking Statements

Materials on this website may contain information that includes or is based upon "forward looking statements" within the meaning of Section 27A of the Securities Act of 1933 and Section 21B of the Securities Exchange Act of 1934.

7

Forward-looking statements are expressions of expectations or forecasts of future events. You can identify these statements by the fact that they do not relate strictly to historical or current facts. They use words such as "anticipate," "estimate," "expect," "project," "intend," "plan," and "believe," in connection with a description of potential earnings or financial performance.

Any and all forward looking statements here or on any materials on this website are intended to express an opinion of earnings potential. Many factors will be important in determining your actual results and no guarantees are made that you will achieve similar results. No guarantees are made that you will achieve any results from the author's ideas and techniques in these materials.

Benton City Consulting LLC assumes no responsibility for any losses or damages resulting from your use of any link, information, or opportunity contained in this eBook or within any other information disclosed by him in any form whatsoever.

Testimonials & Examples

Testimonials and examples on this website may not reflect the typical purchaser's experience and are not intended to represent or guarantee that anyone will achieve the same or similar results.

There is no assurance that you will do as well using the same information or strategies as set forth on the website. If you rely on specific income or earnings figures, you accept all risk. Your financial results are likely to differ from those described in the testimonials.

COPYRIGHT WARNING: The legal notices and administrative pages on this website, including this one, have been drafted by the Law Offices of Douglas Slain in October, 2012. **Benton City Consulting LLC** has paid to license the use of these legal notices and administrative pages for your protection and ours. This material may not be used in any way for any reason; unauthorized use is policed via Copyscape to detect violators.

QUESTIONS/COMMENTS/CONCERNS: If you have any questions about the contents of this page, or simply wish to reach us for any other reason, you may do so by using our Contact information.

Benton City Consulting

108 Acord Road

Benton City, WA 99320-

Budpersonal @gmail.com

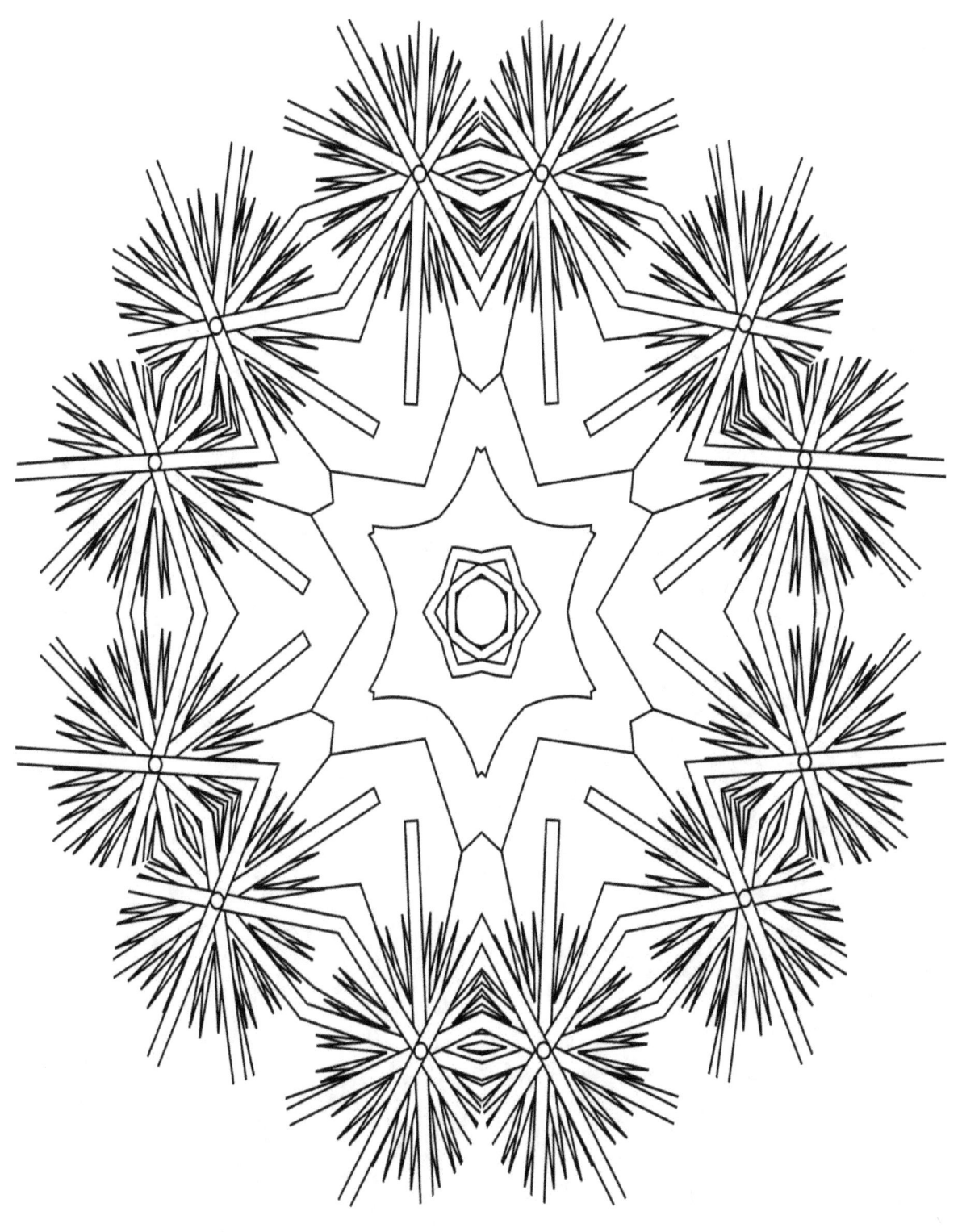

Here is your download link.

Bud's Secret Garden Retreat

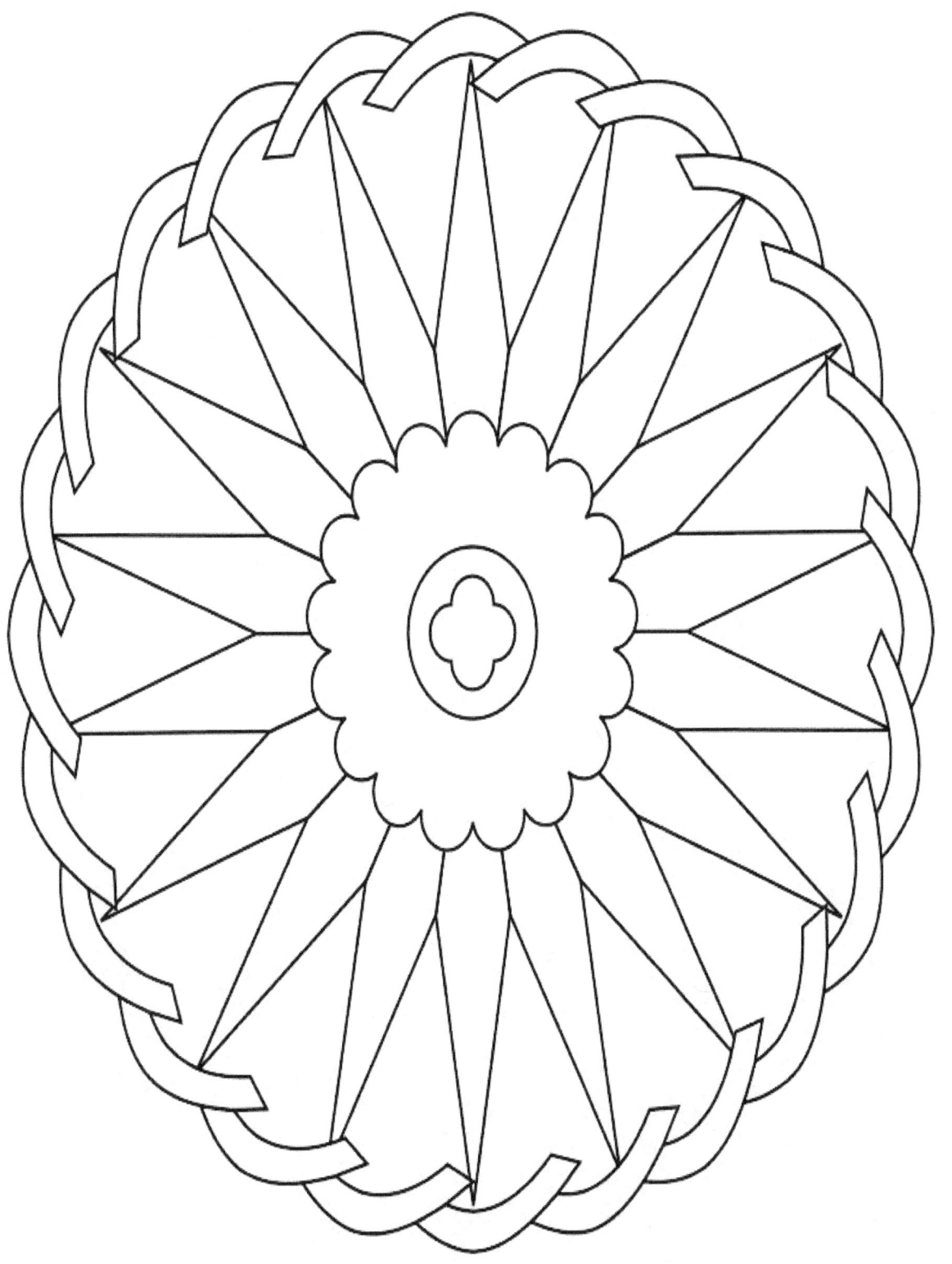

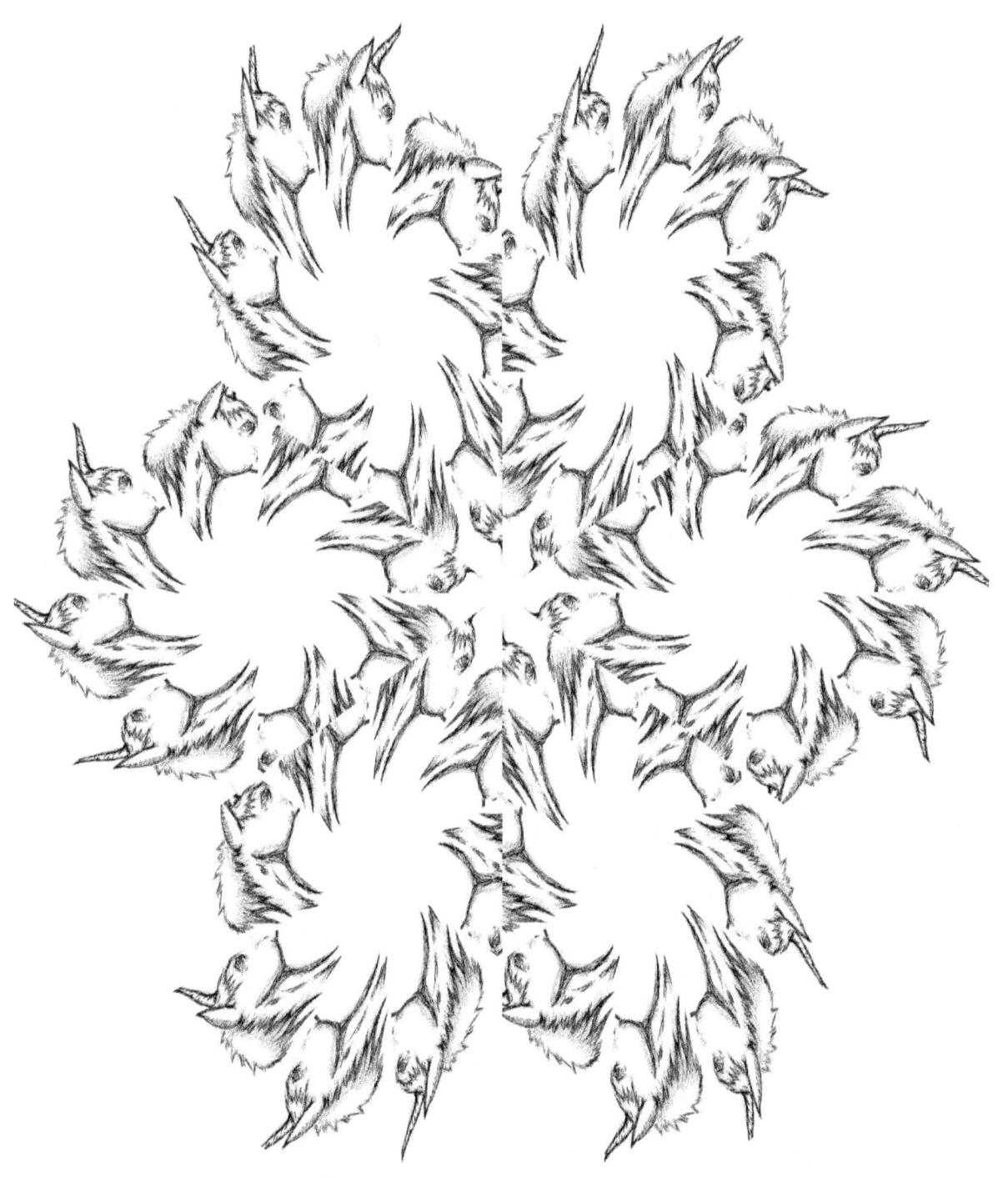

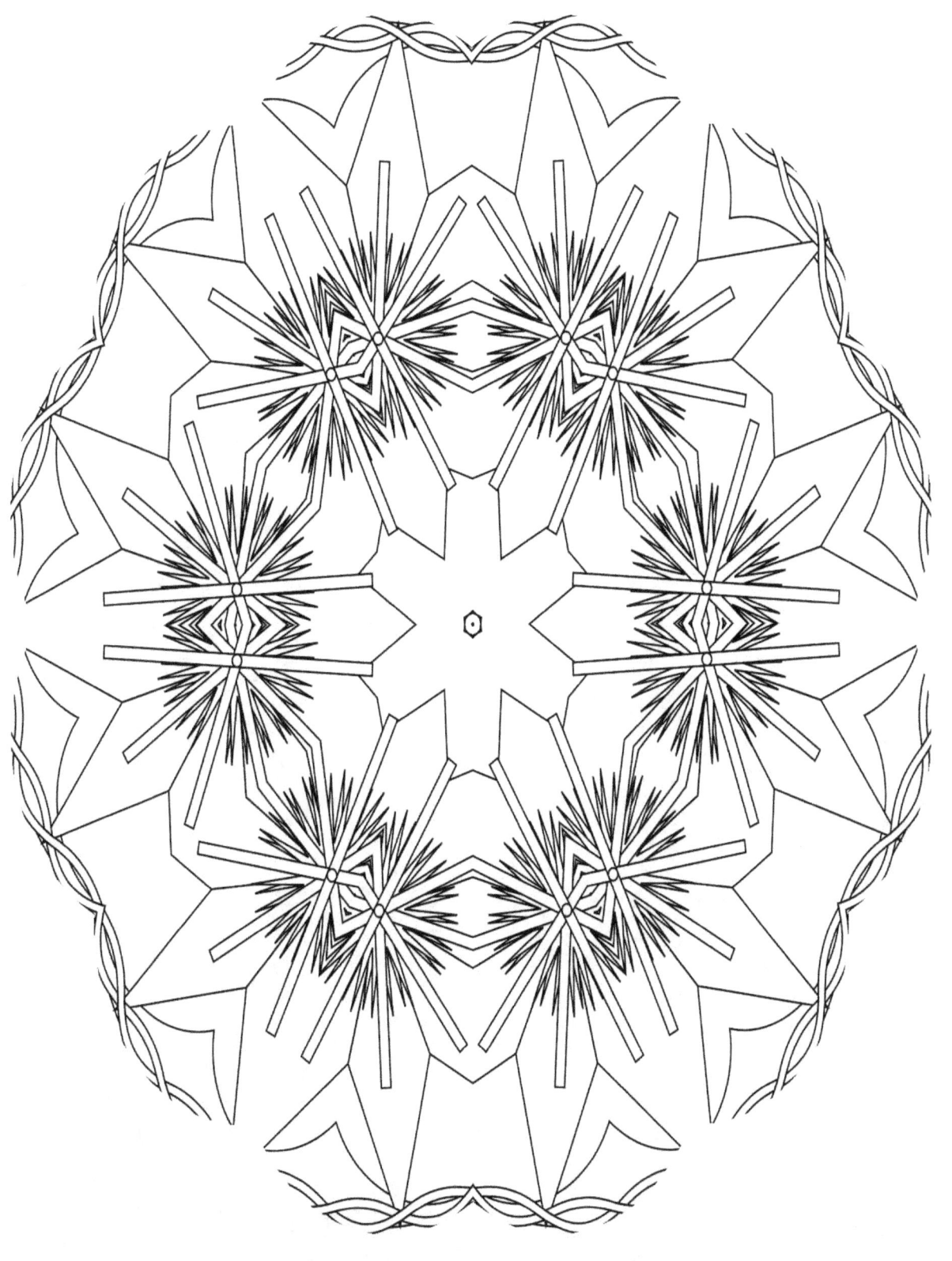

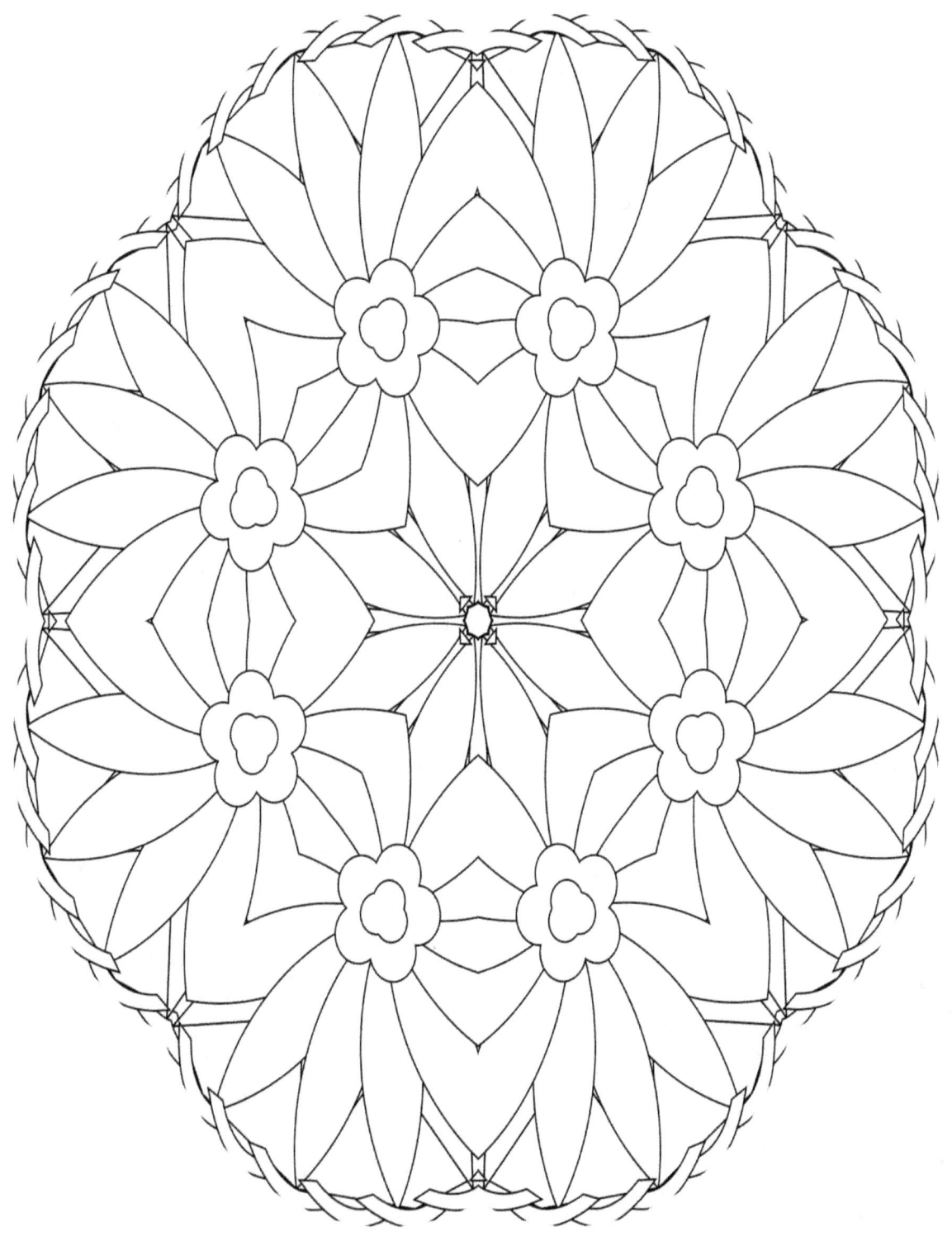

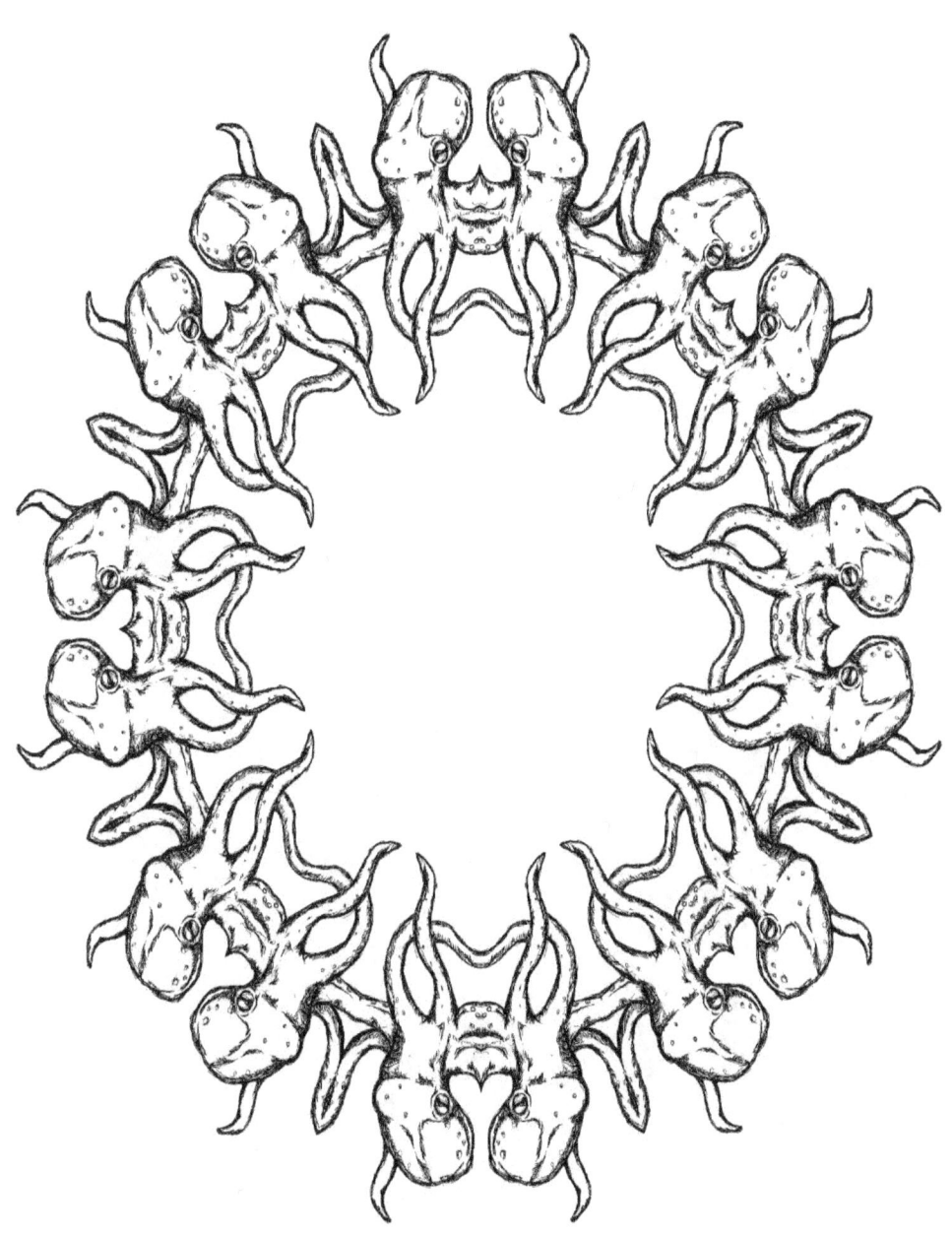

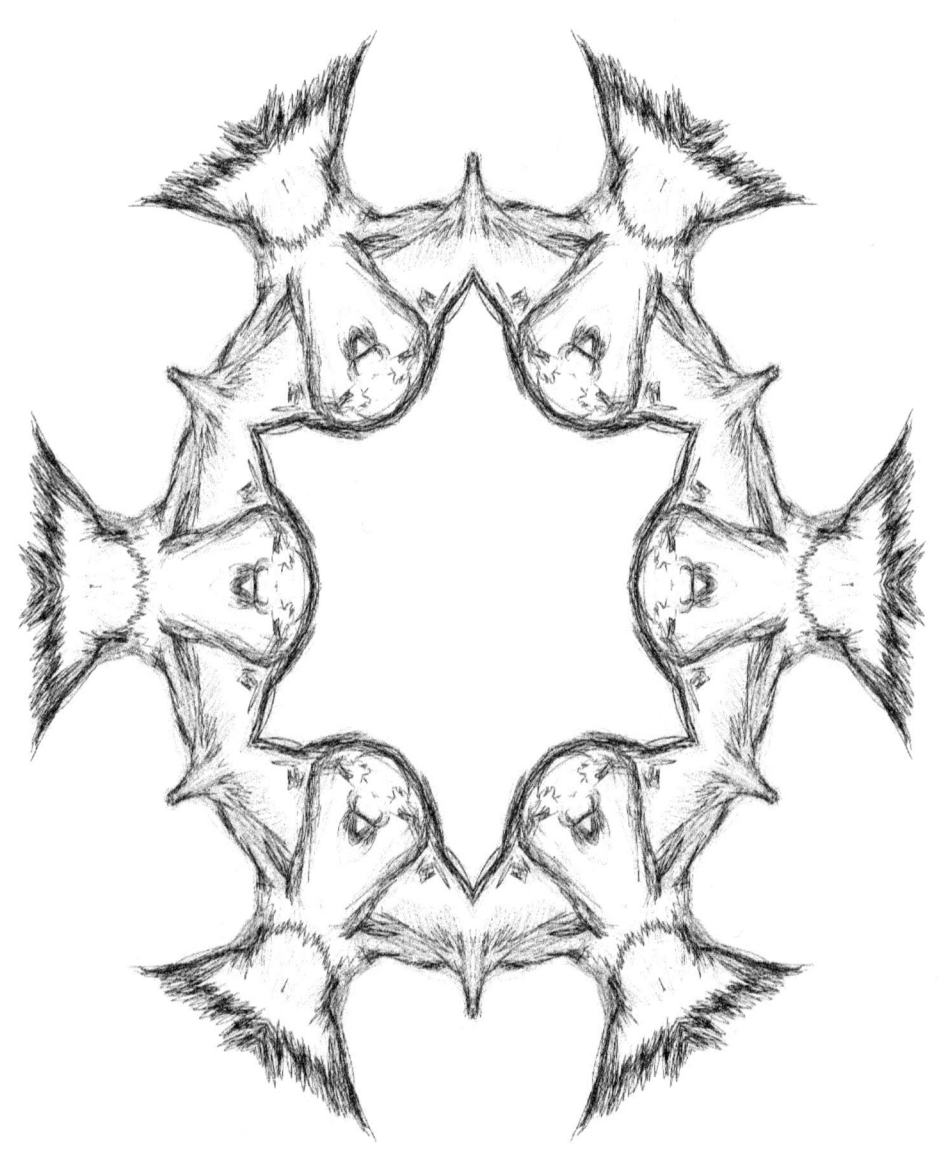

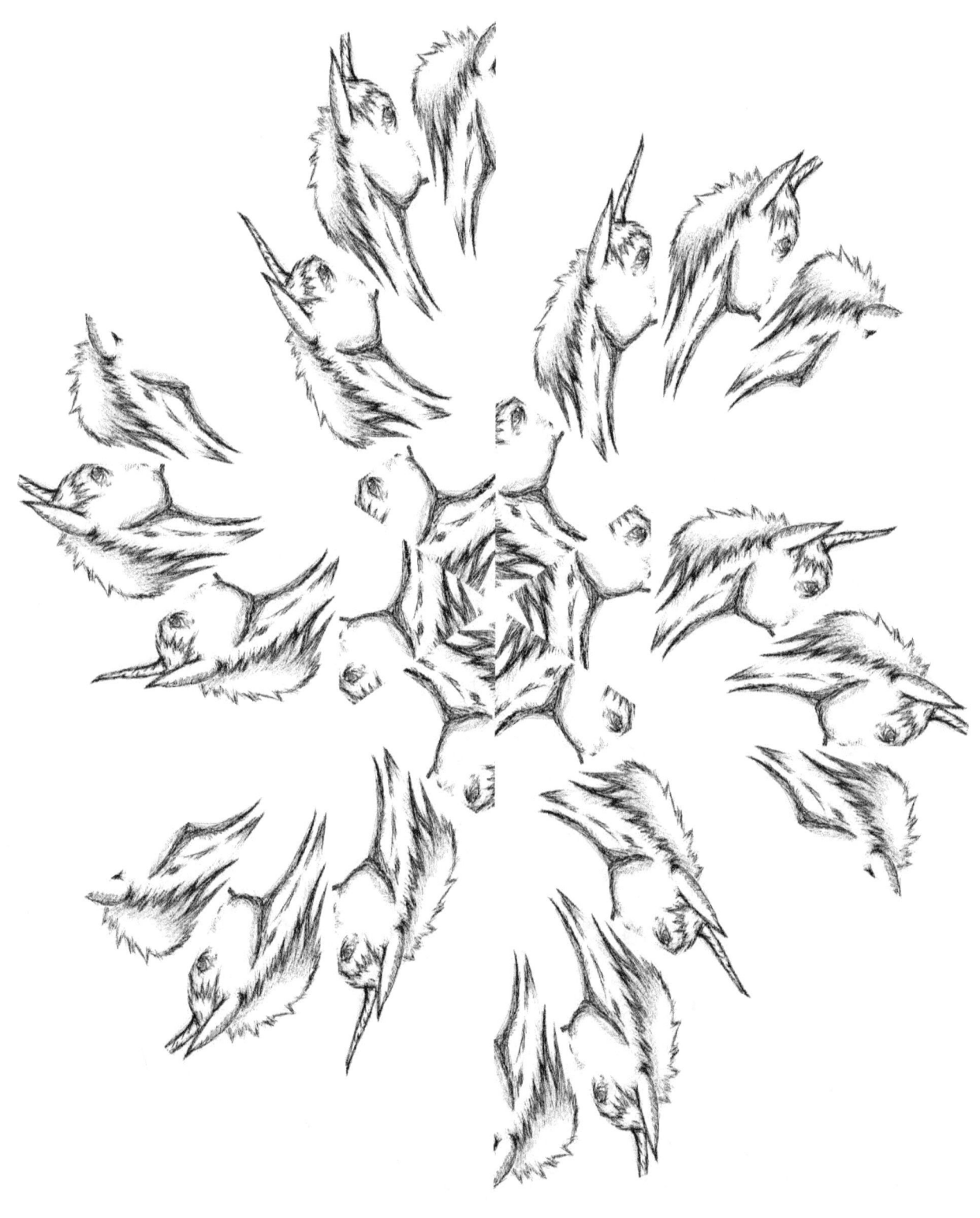

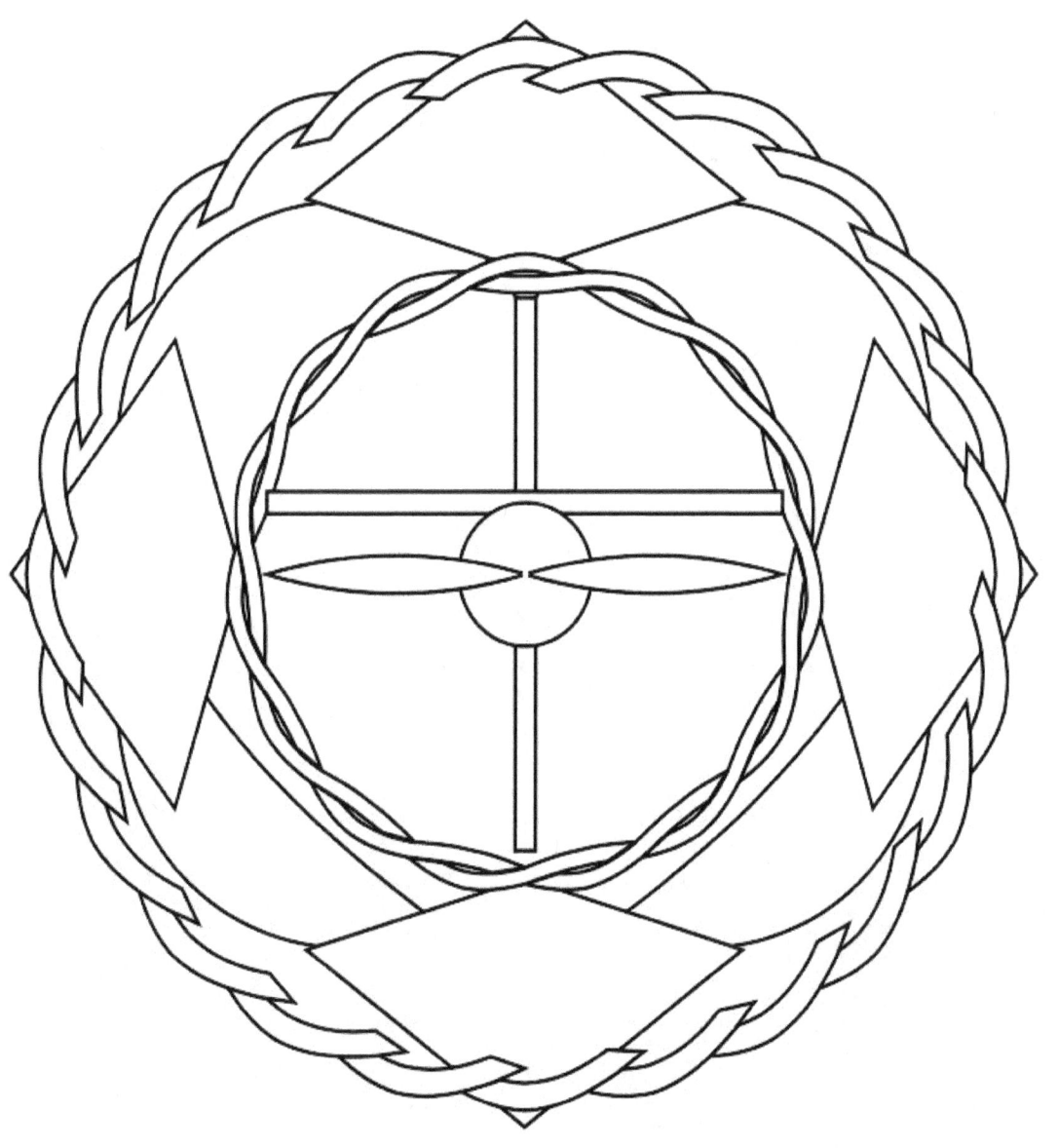

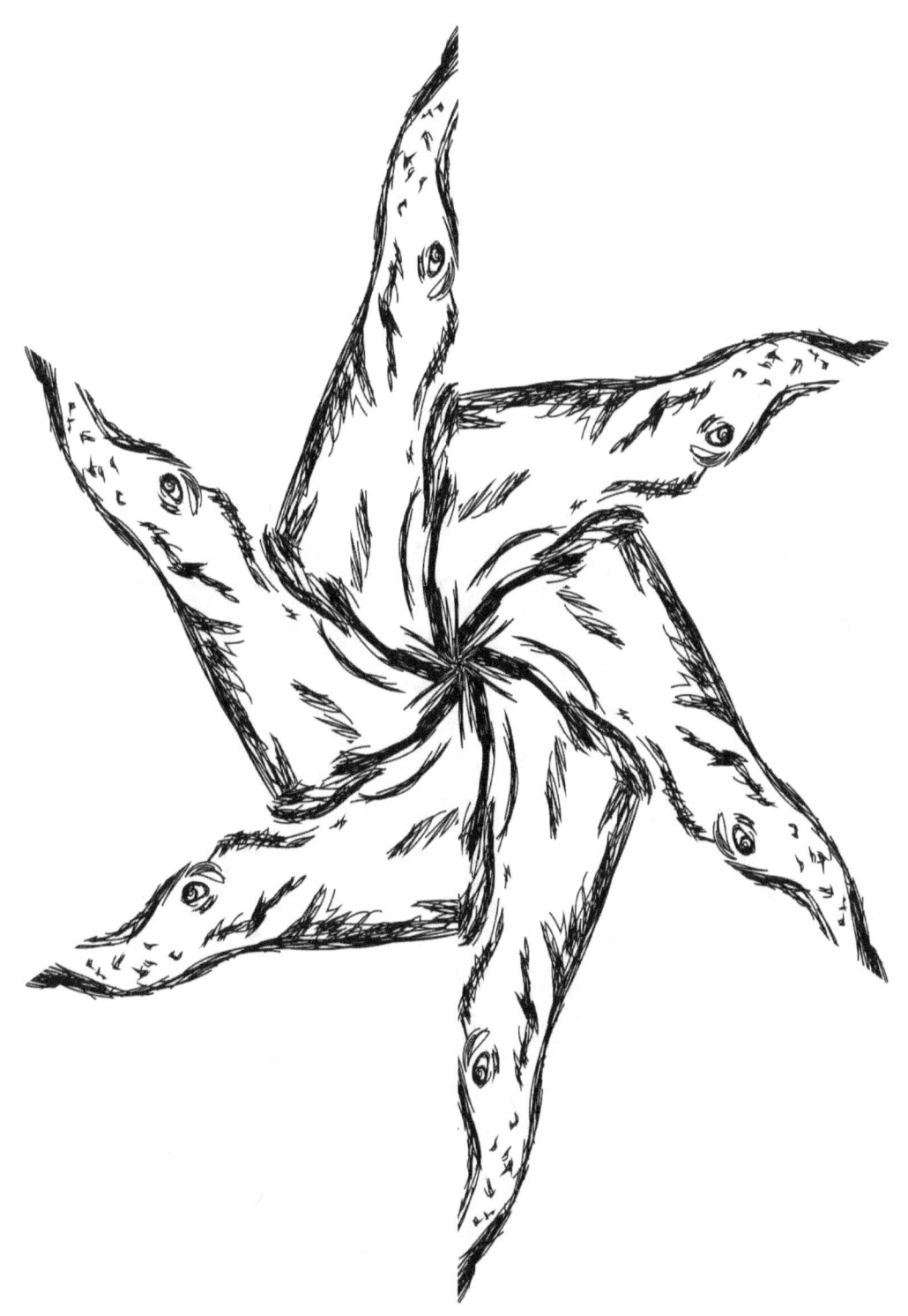

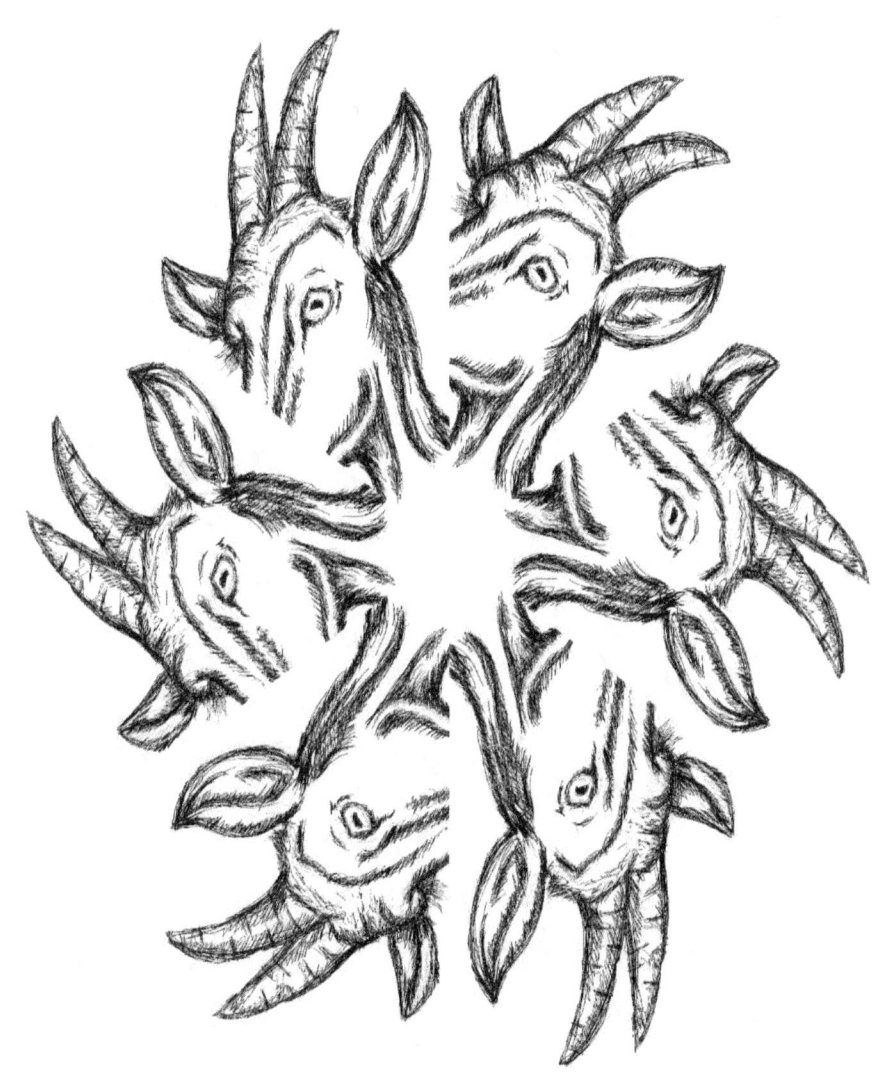

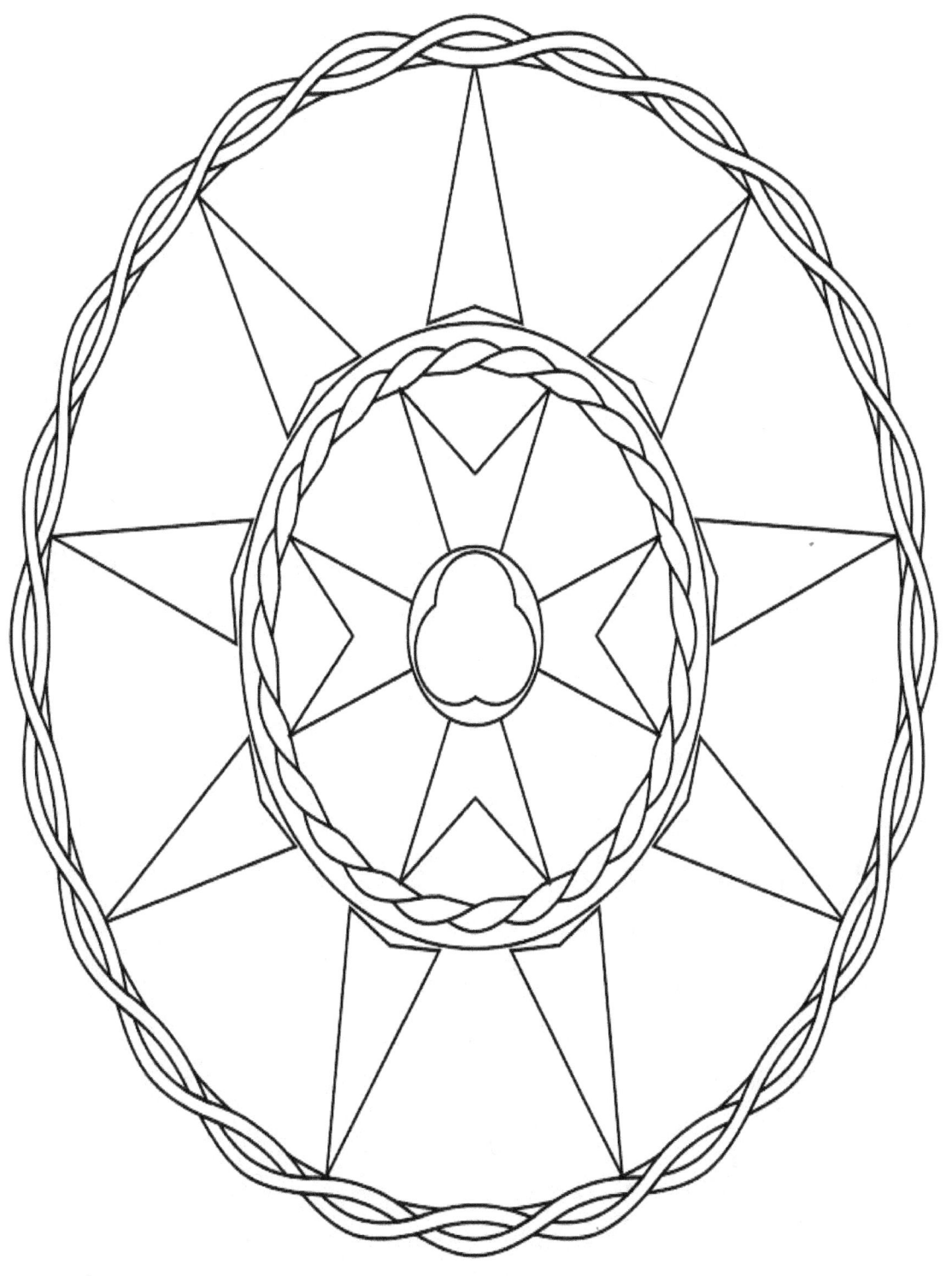

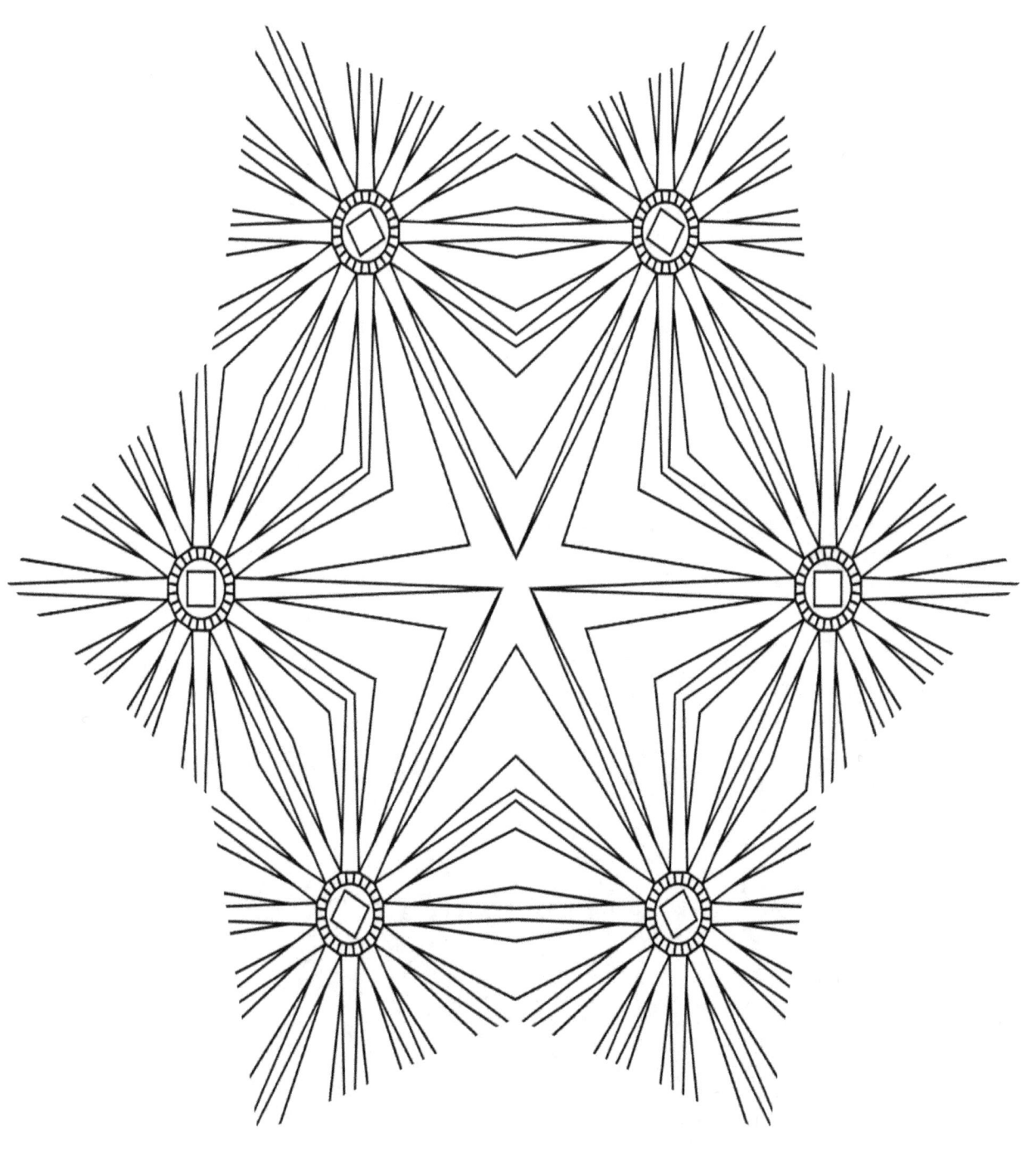

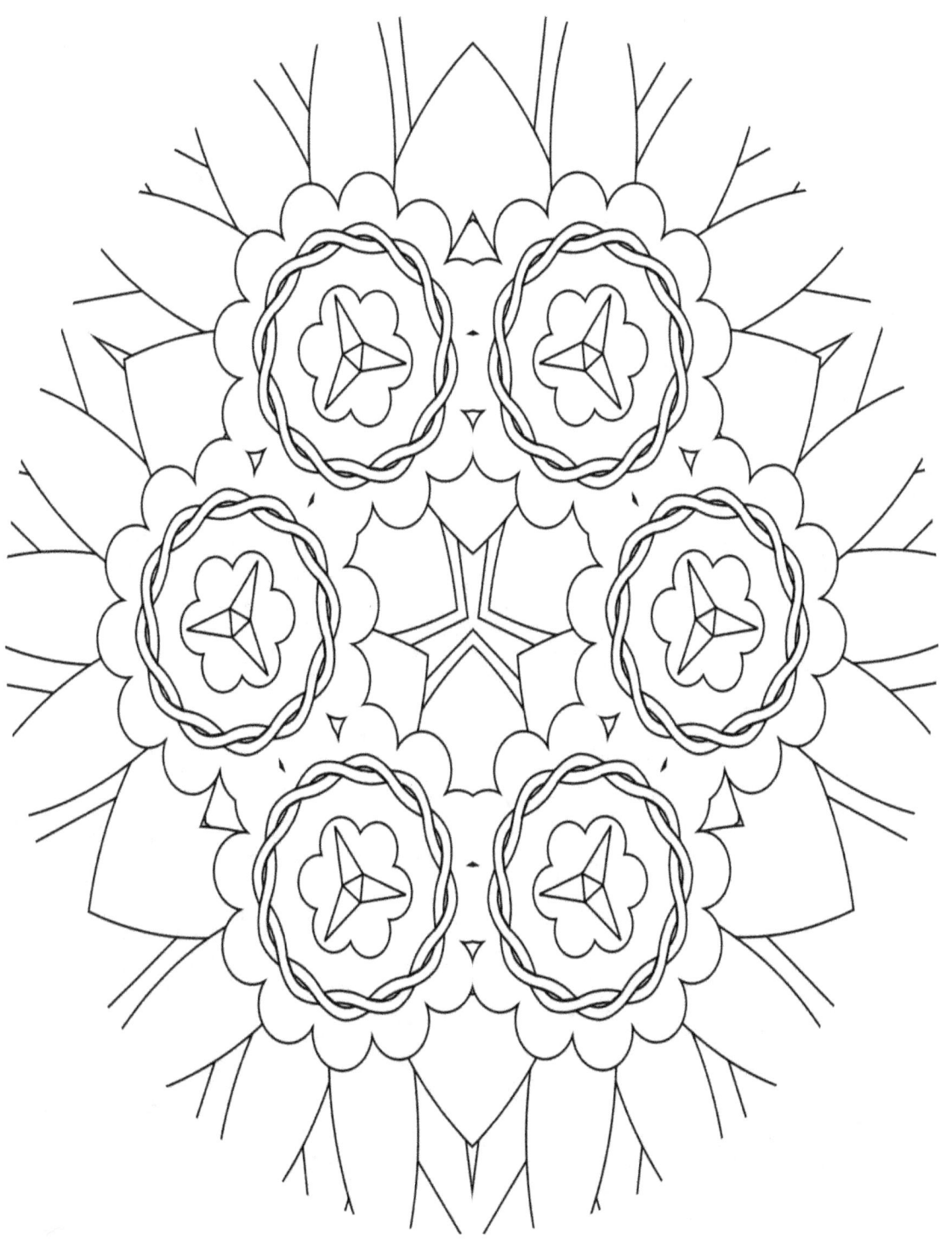

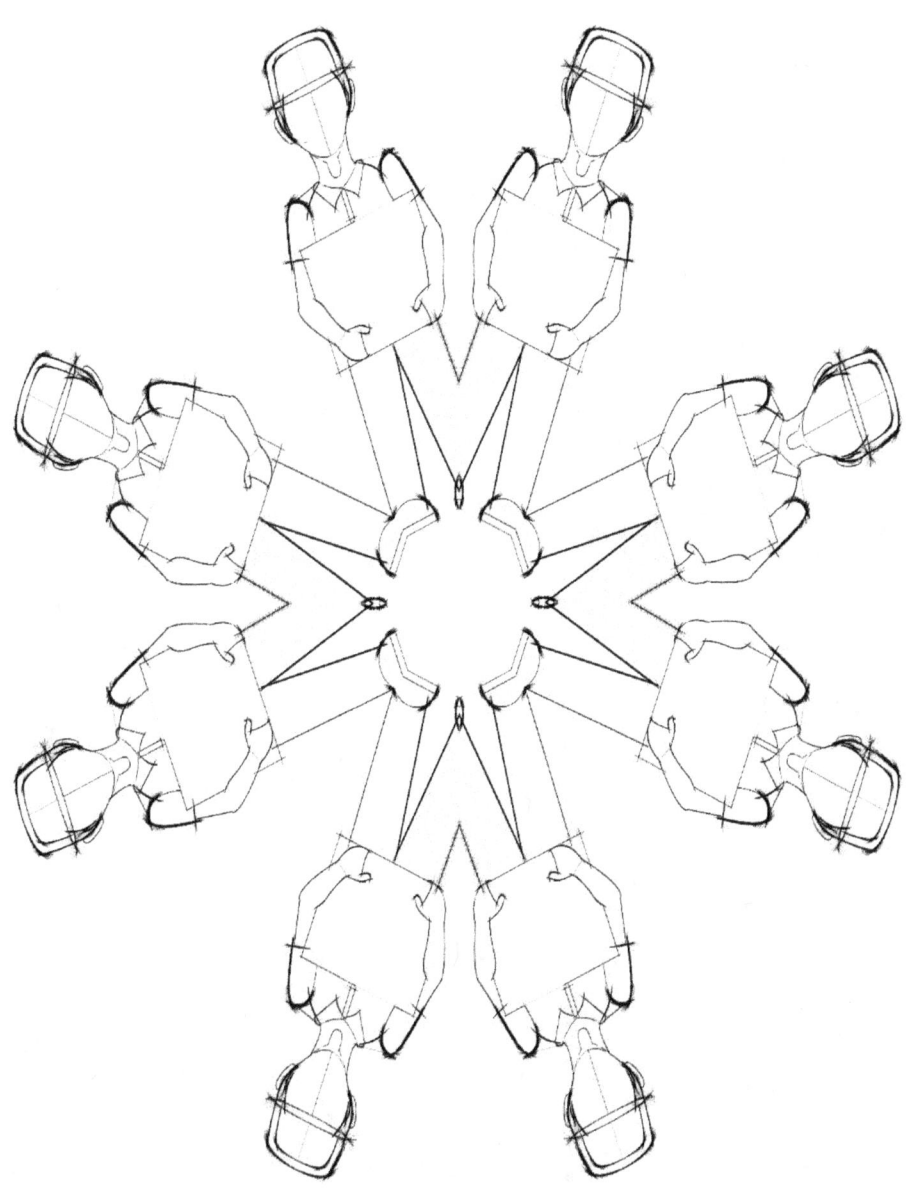

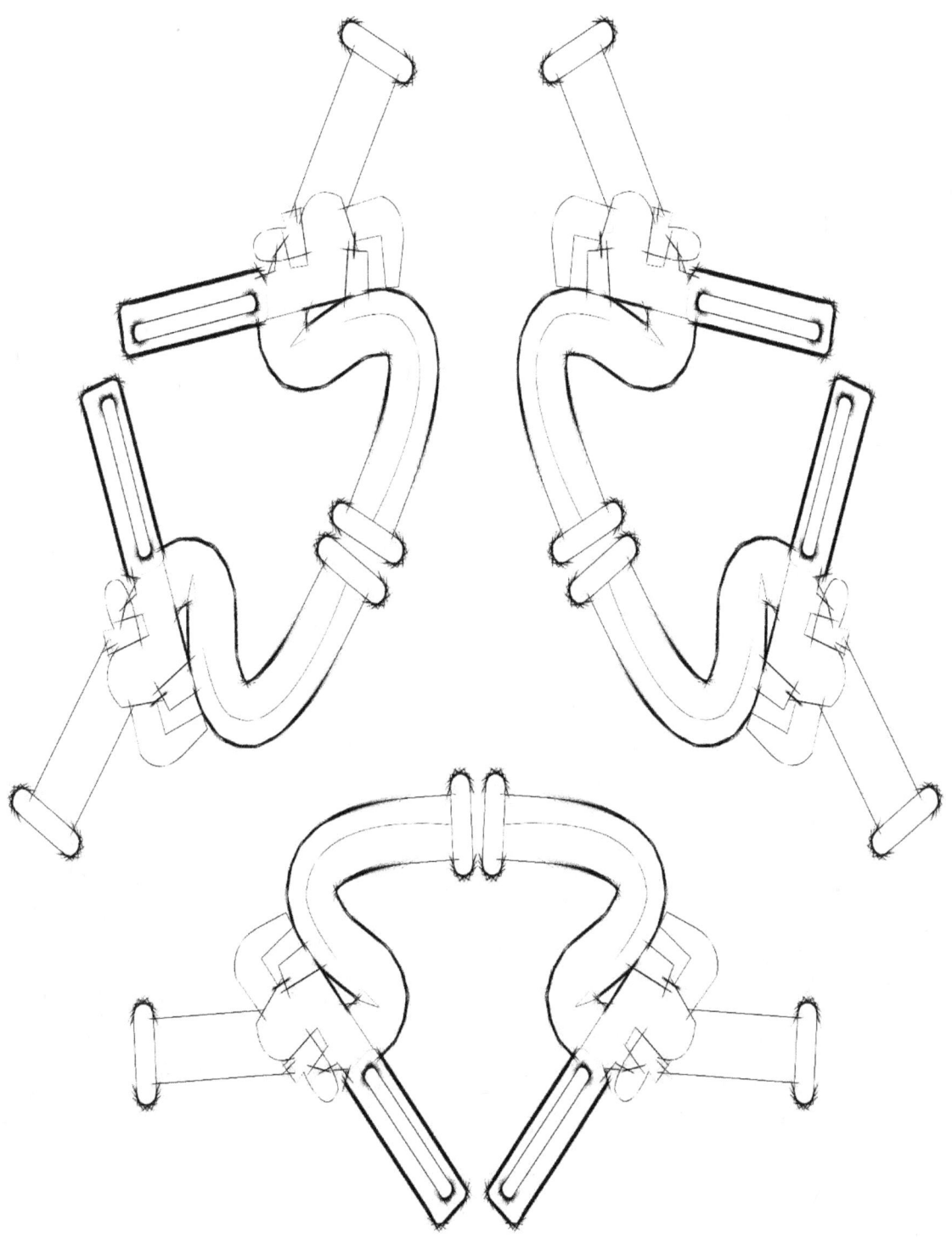

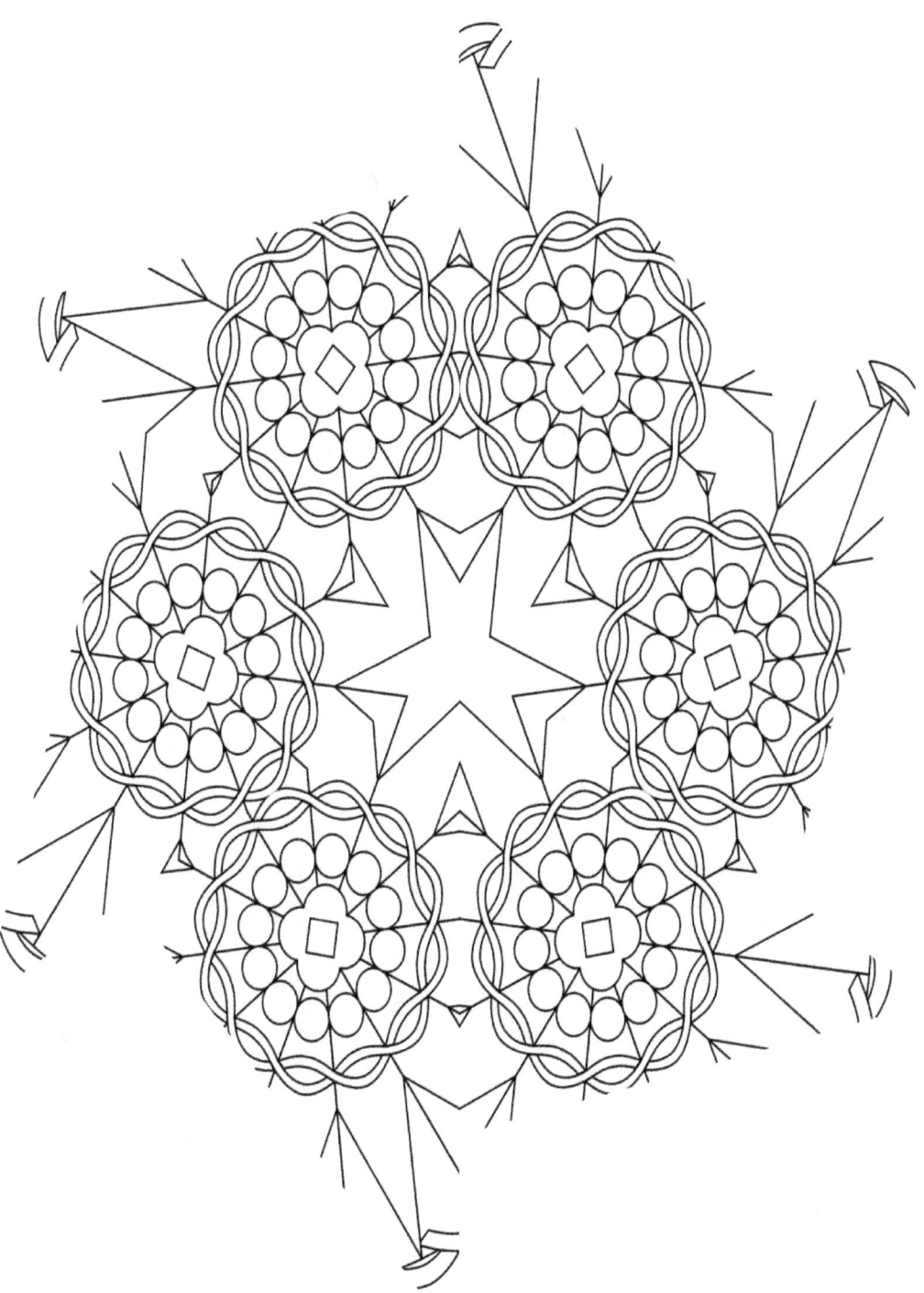

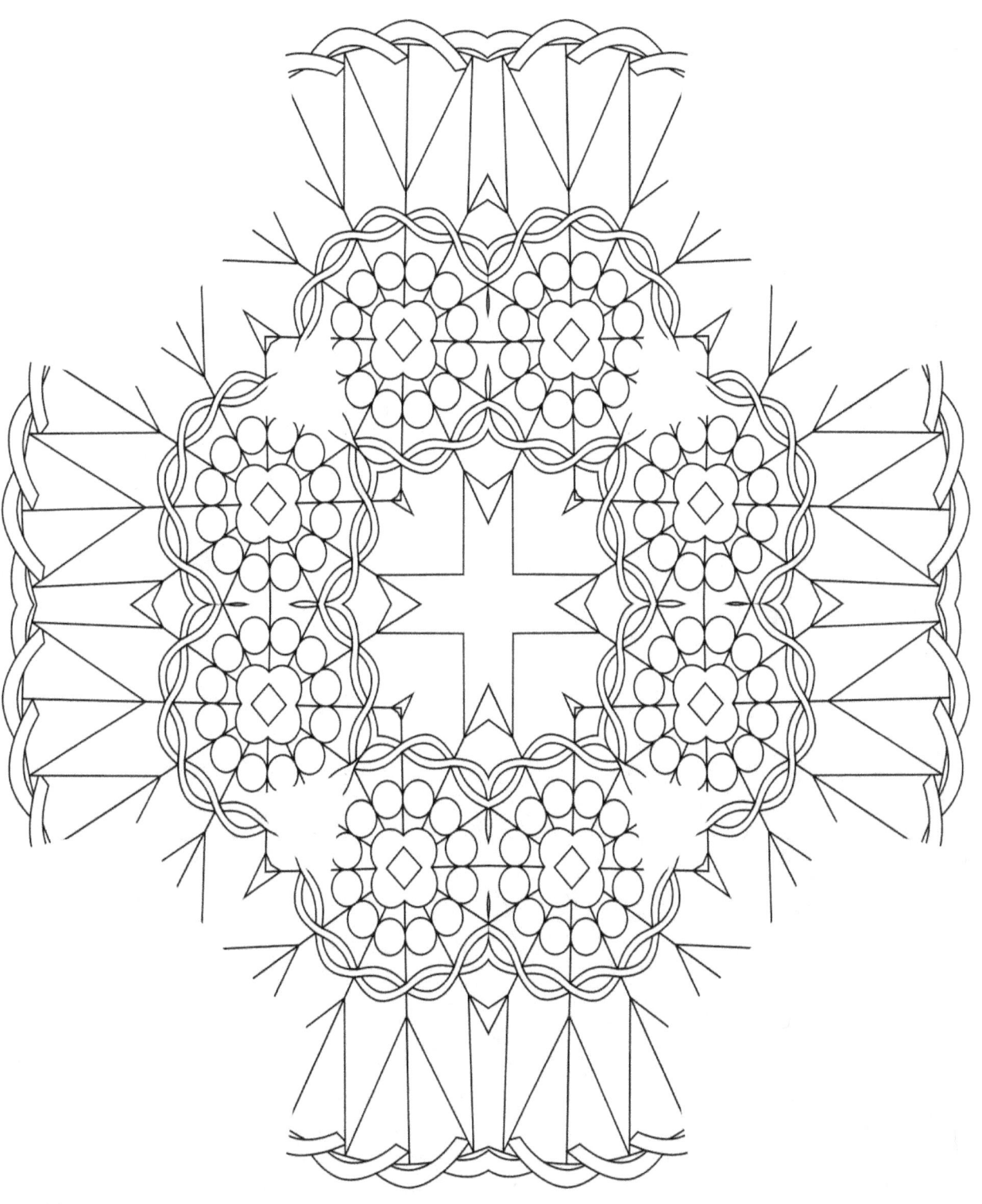

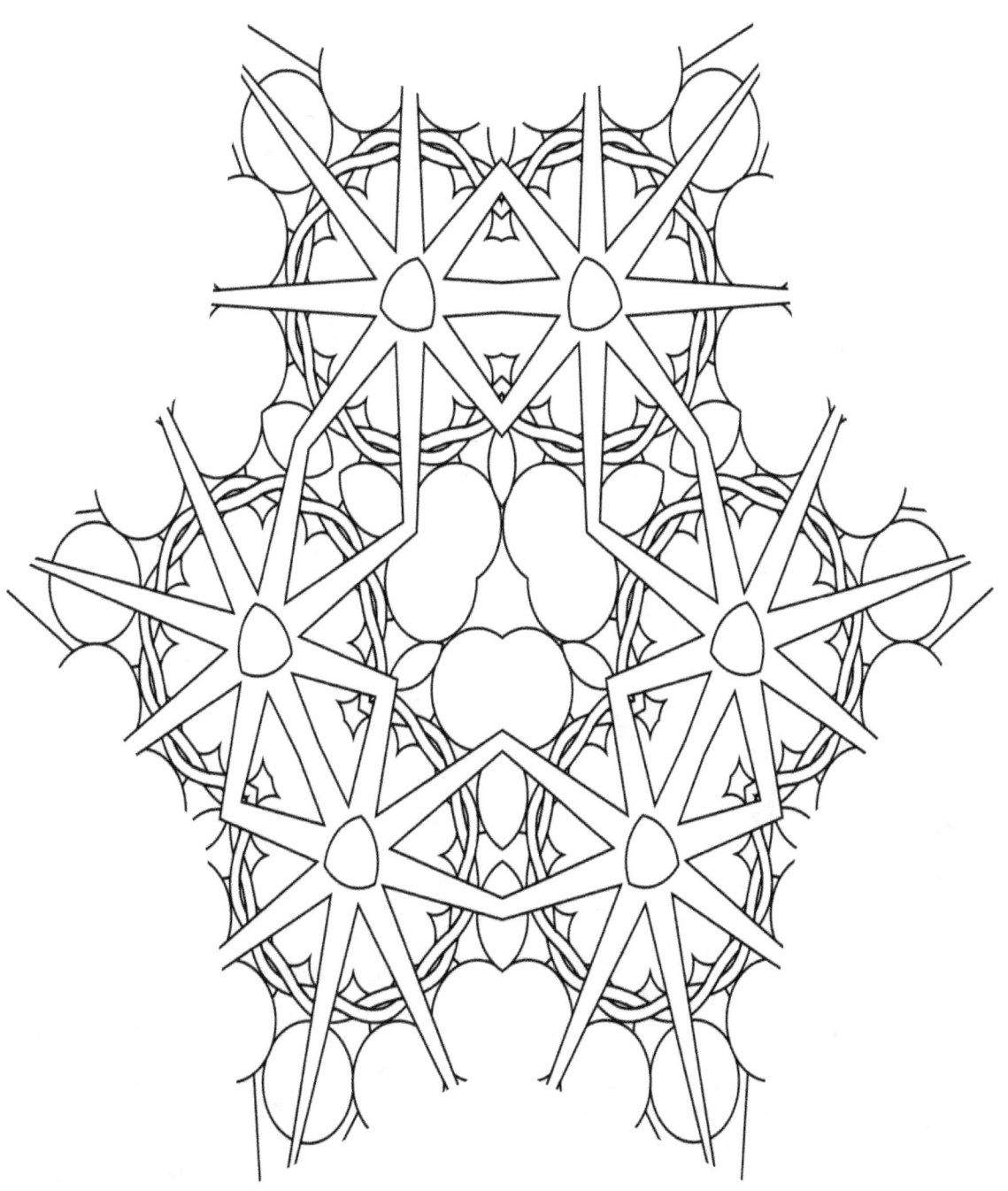

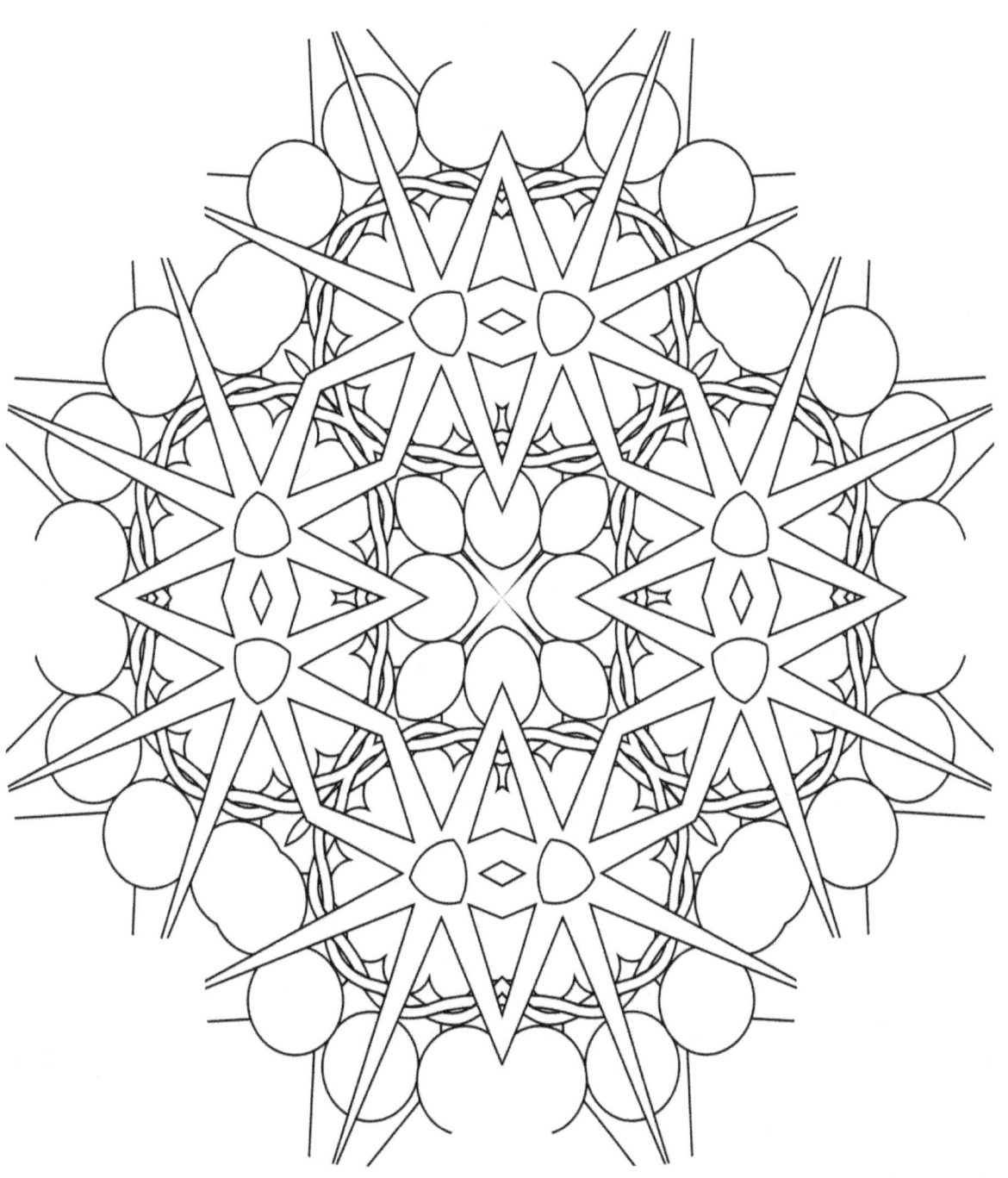

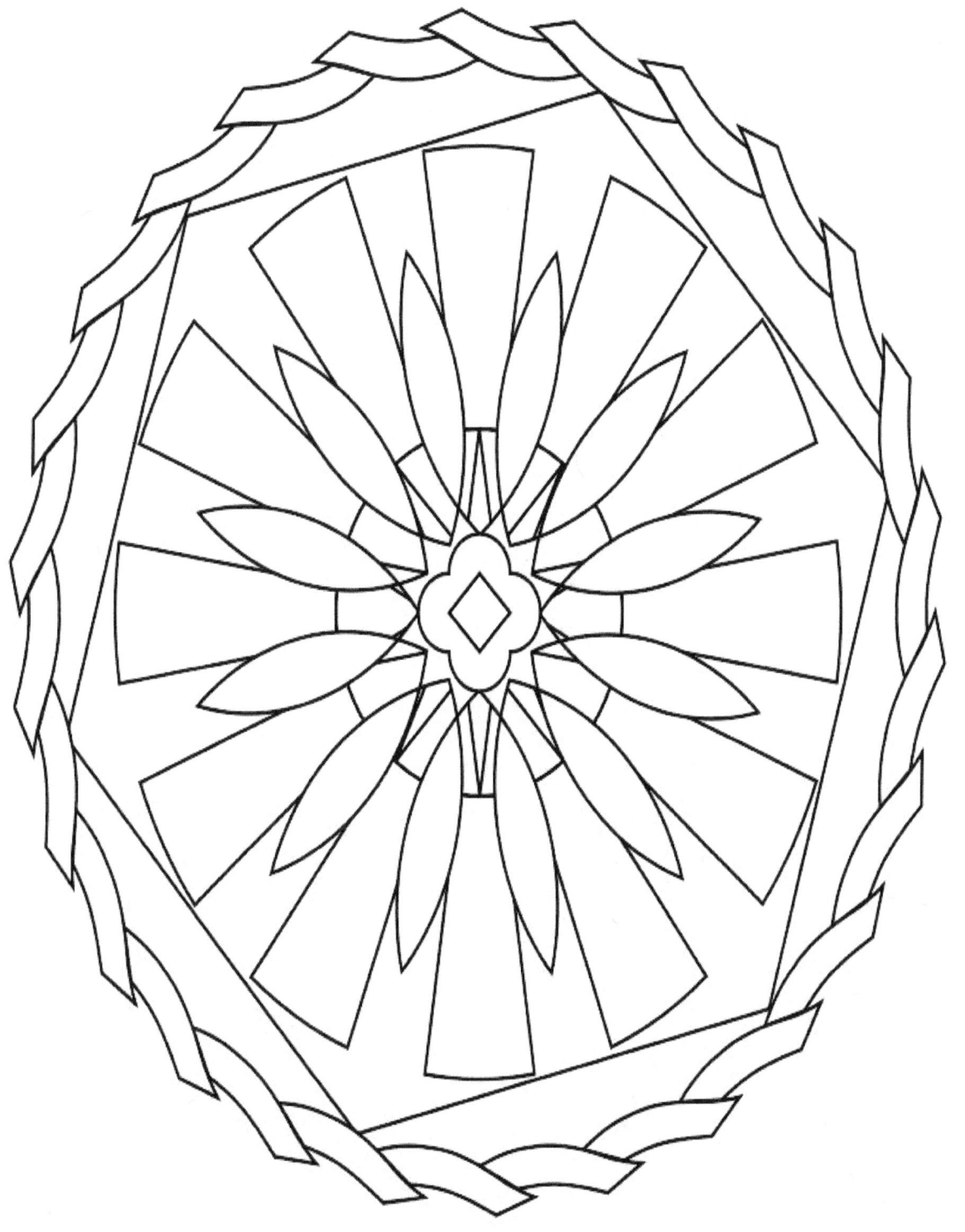

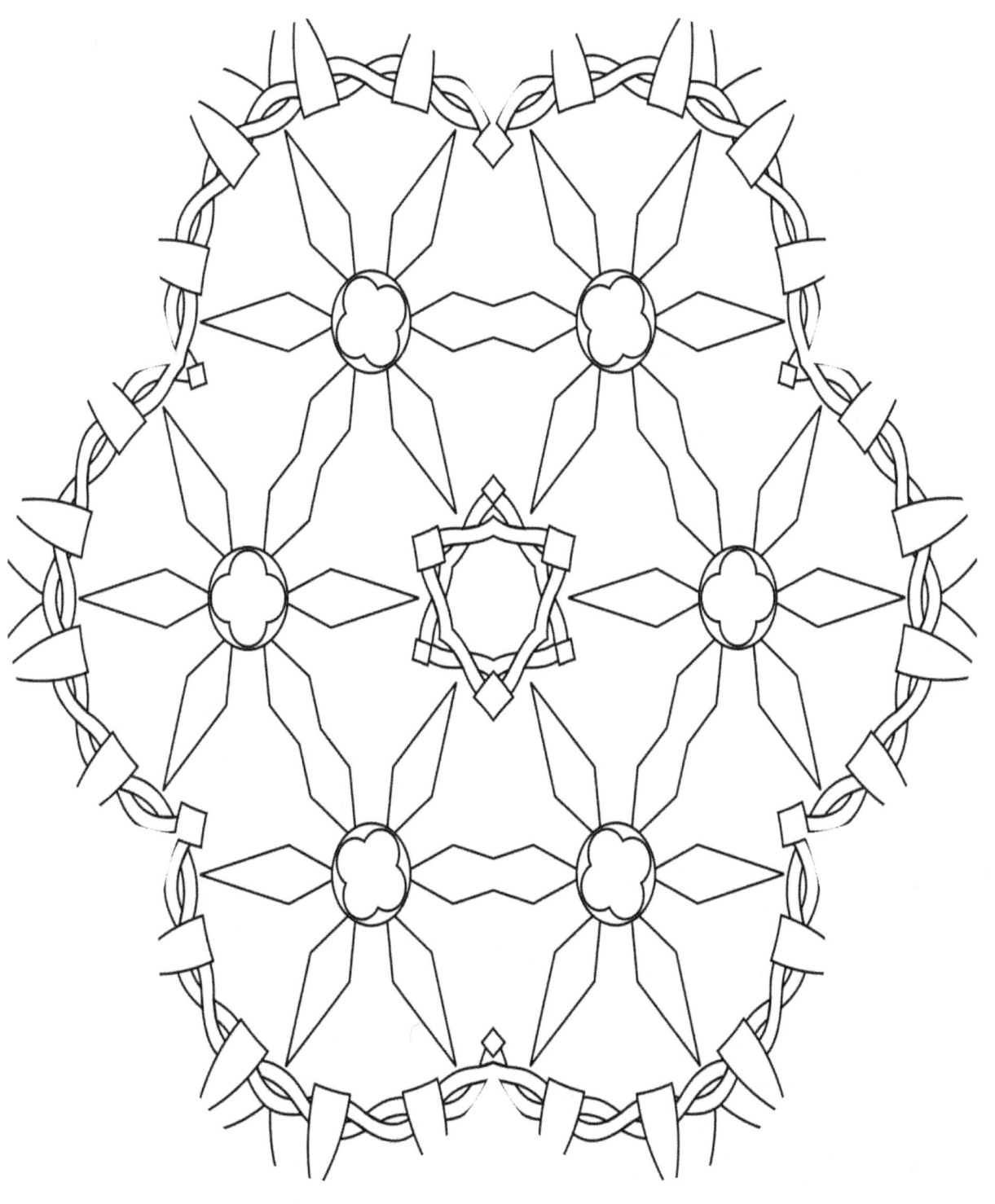

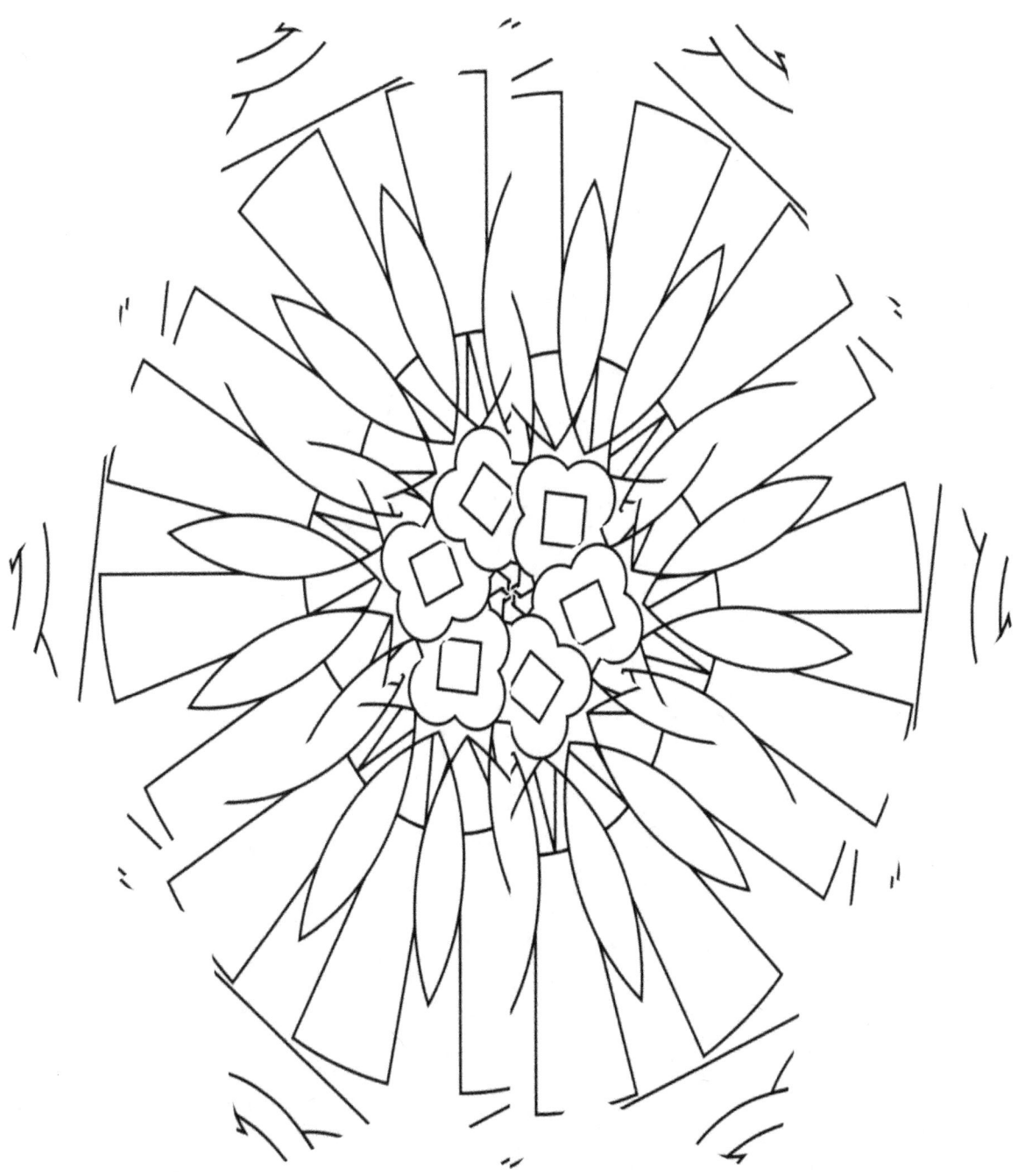

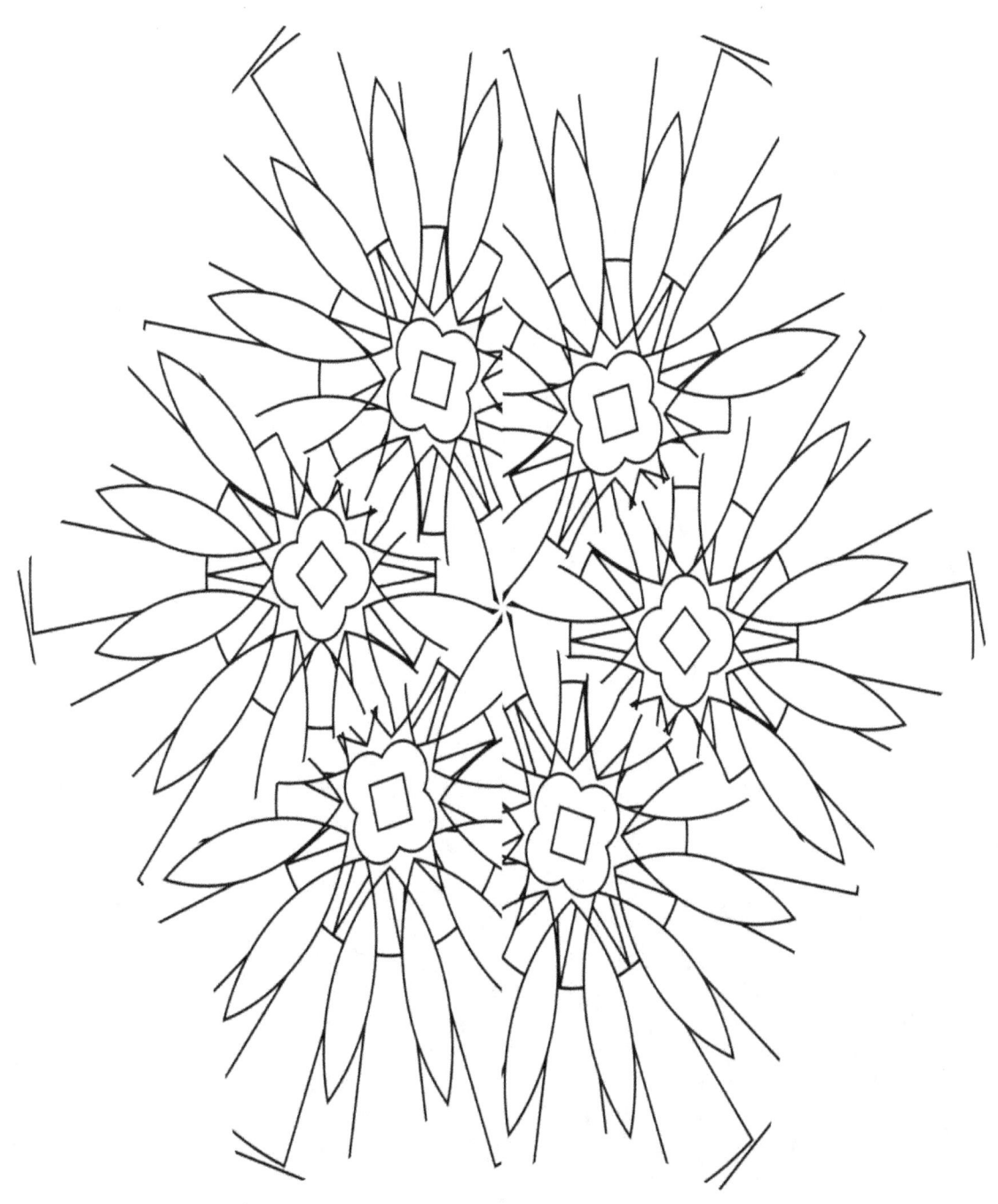

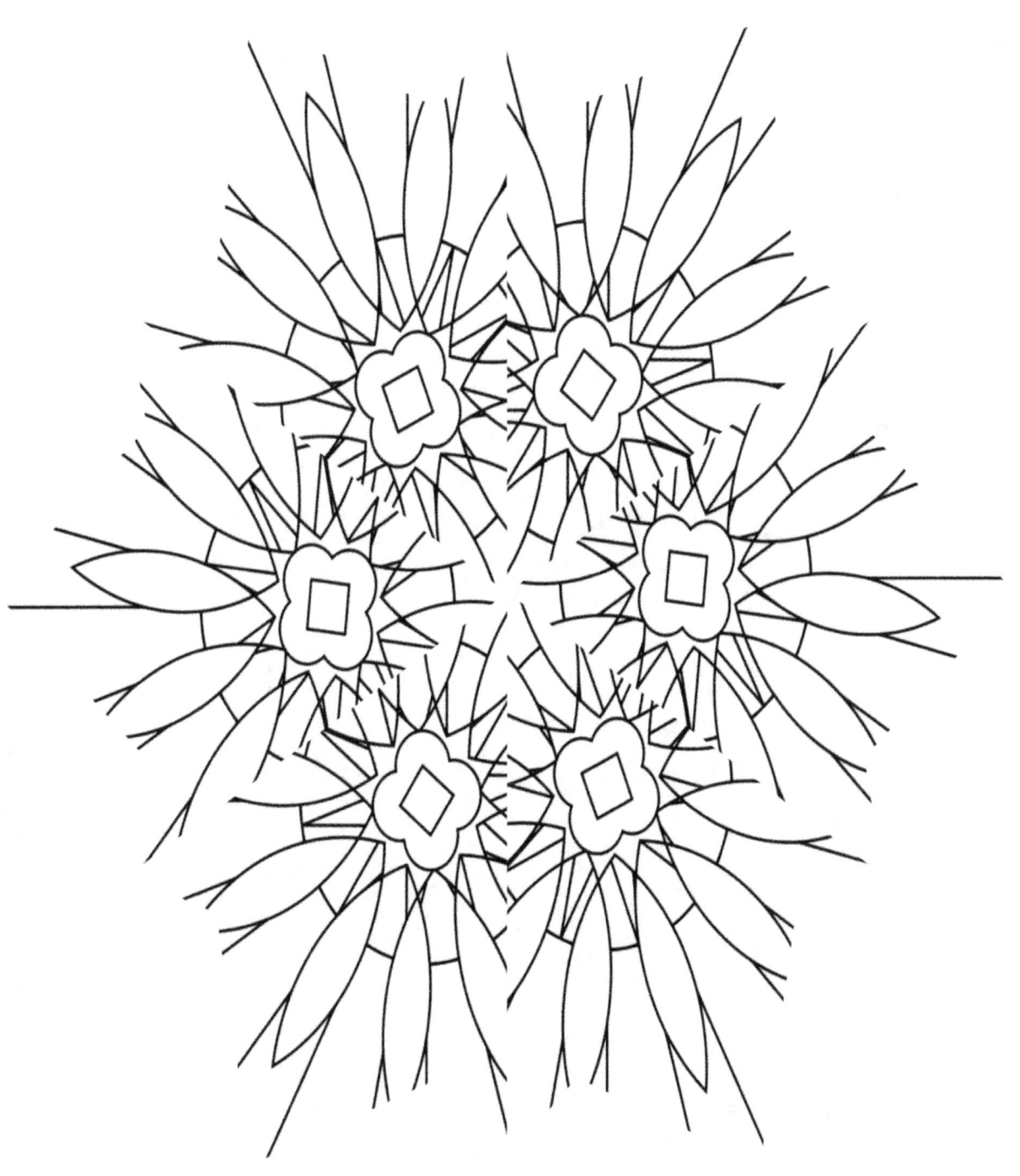

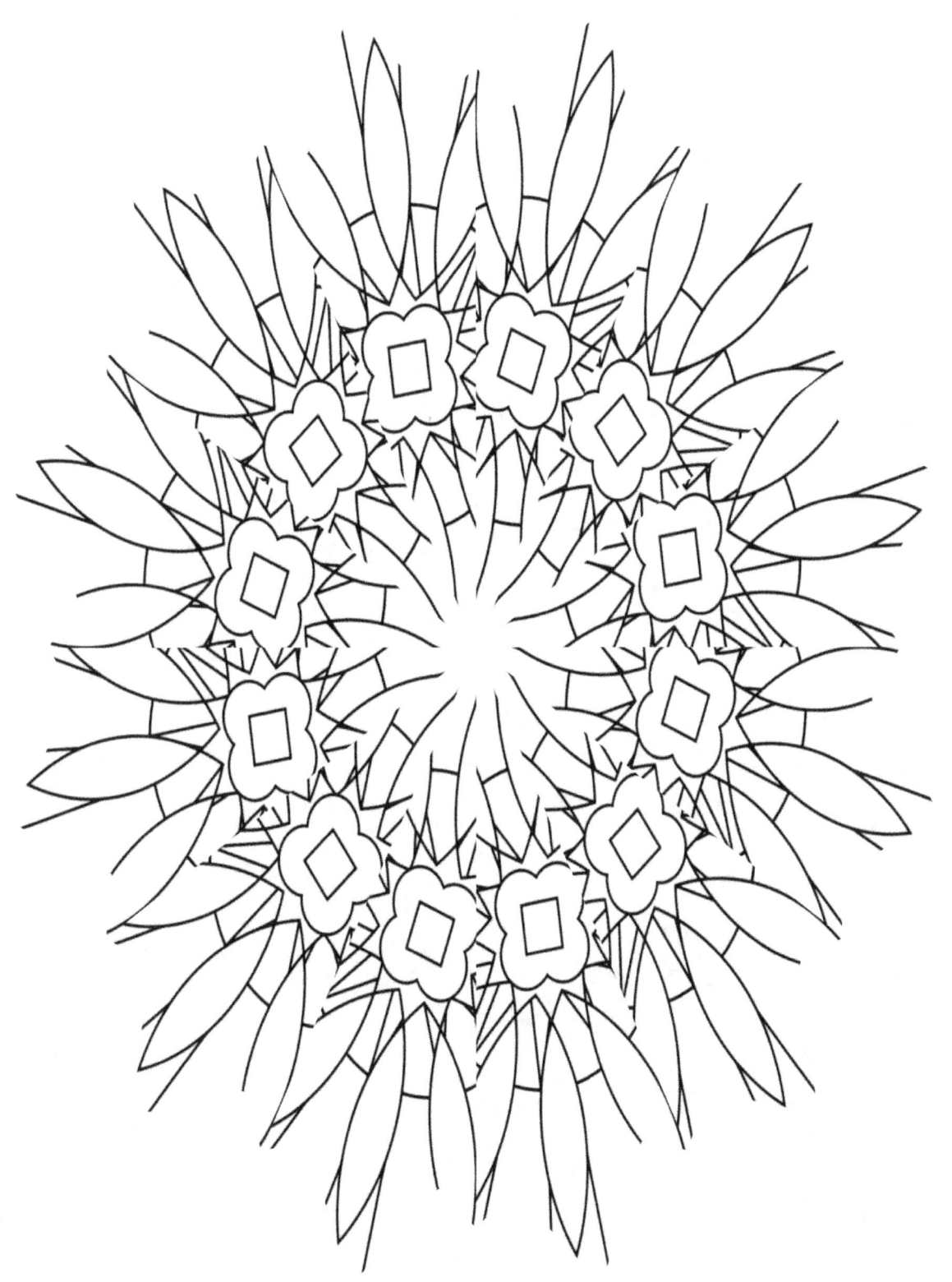

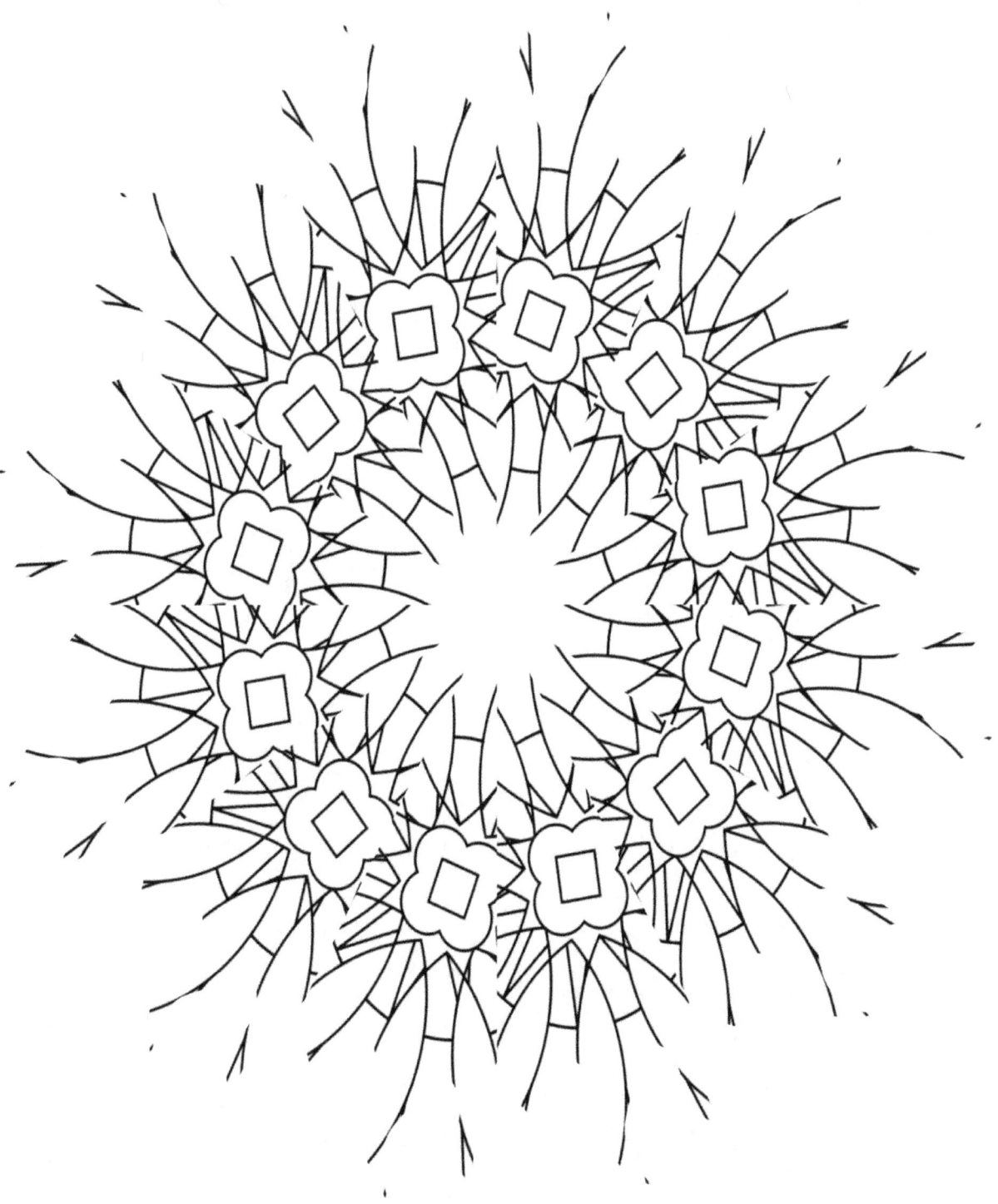

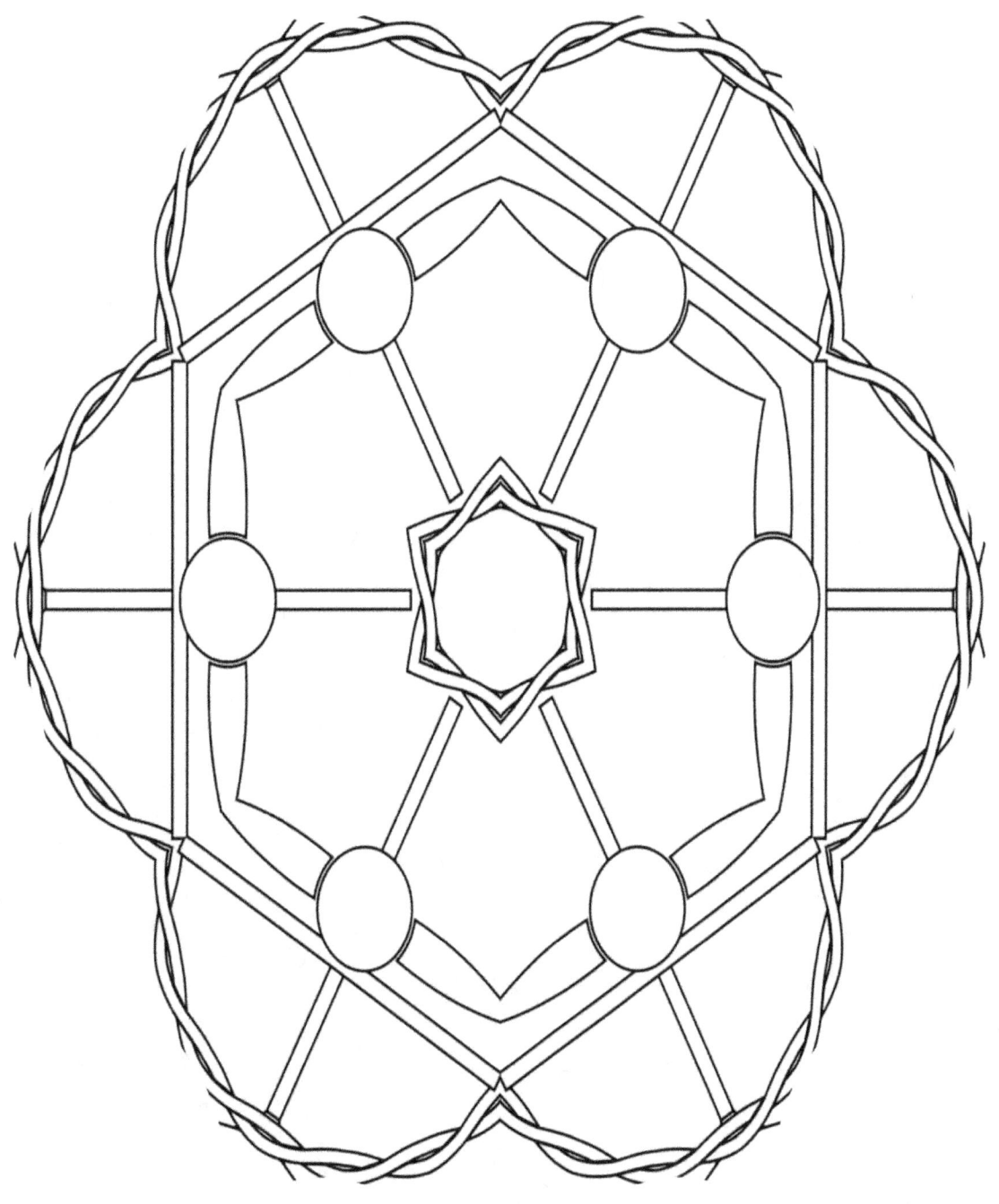

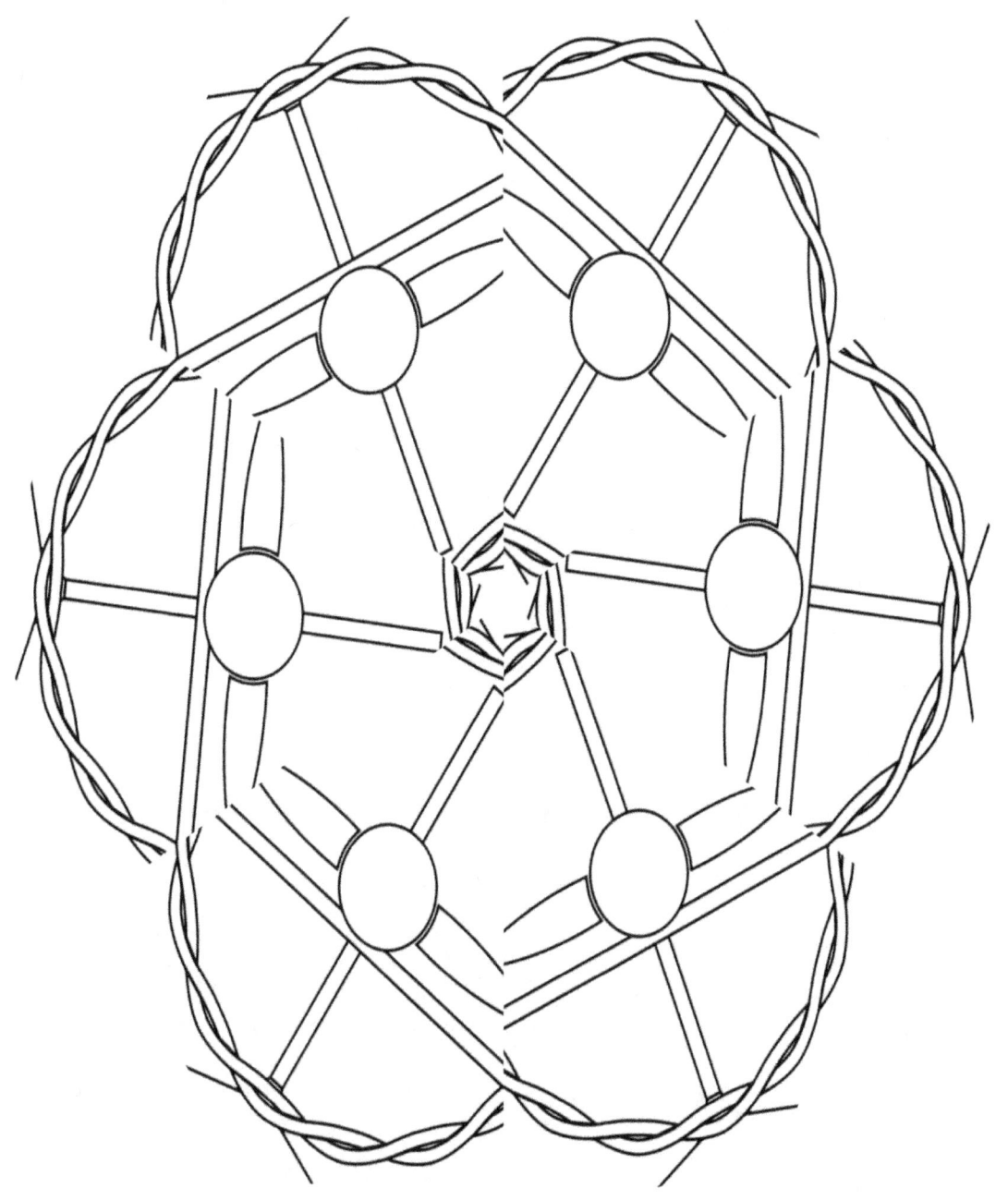

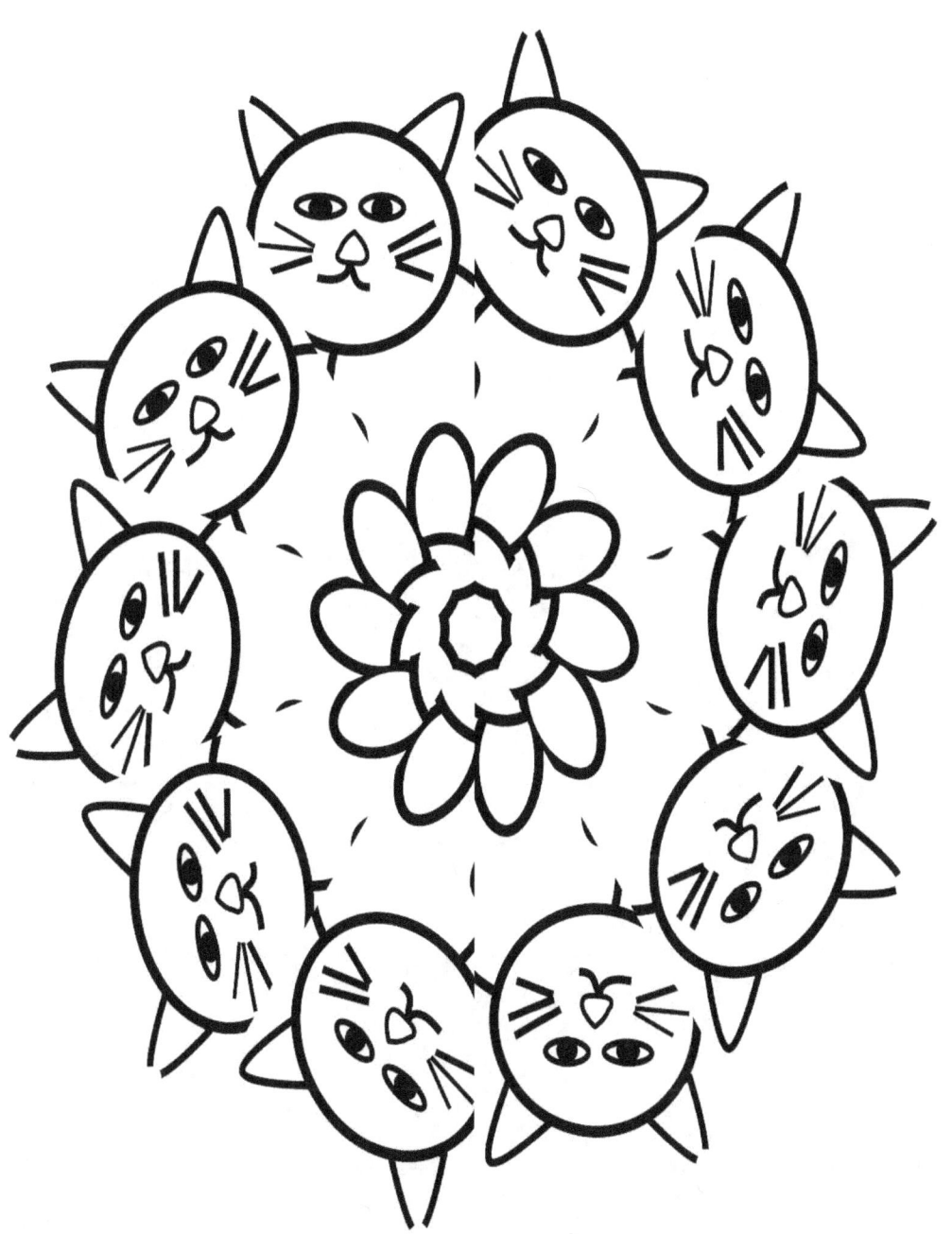

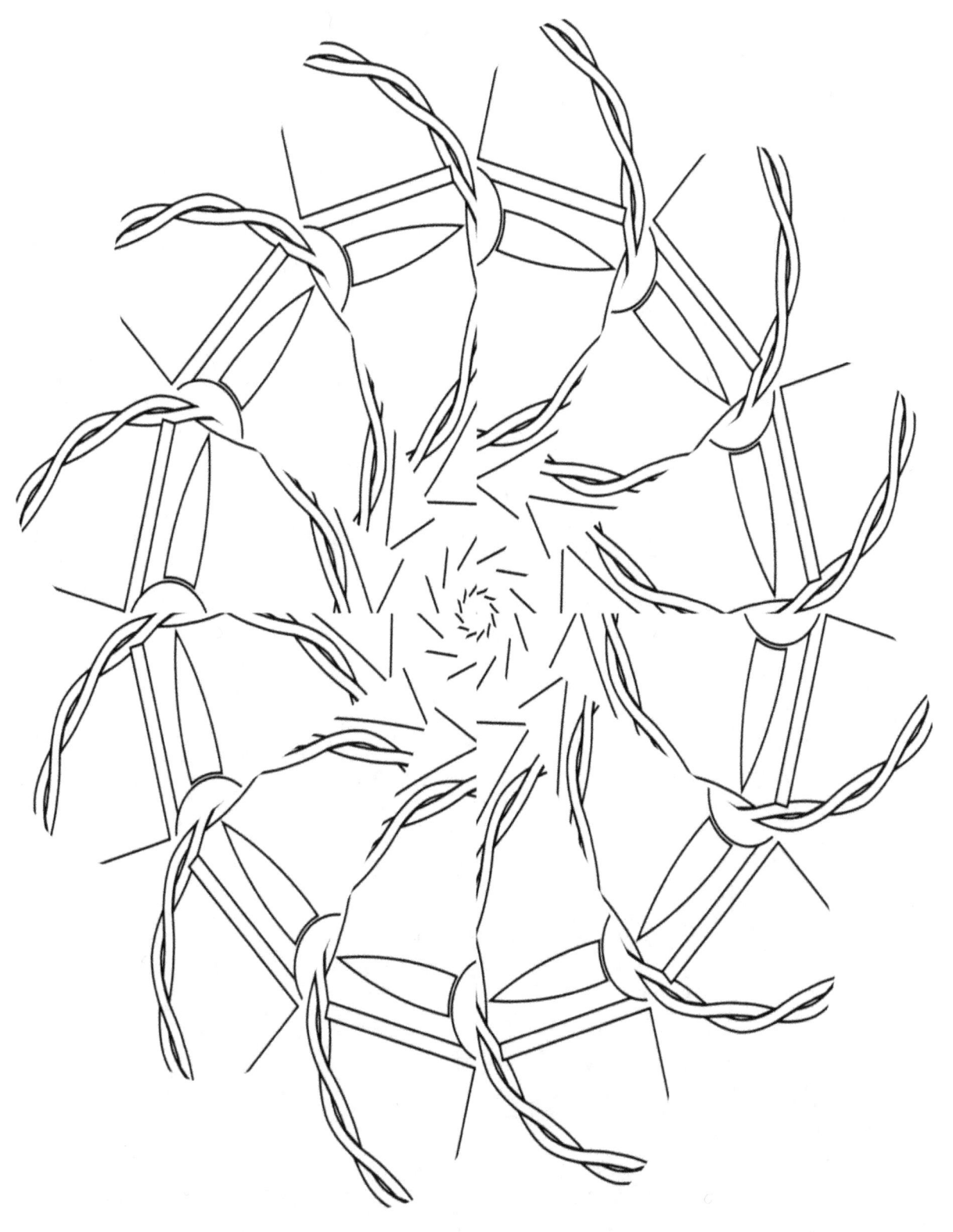

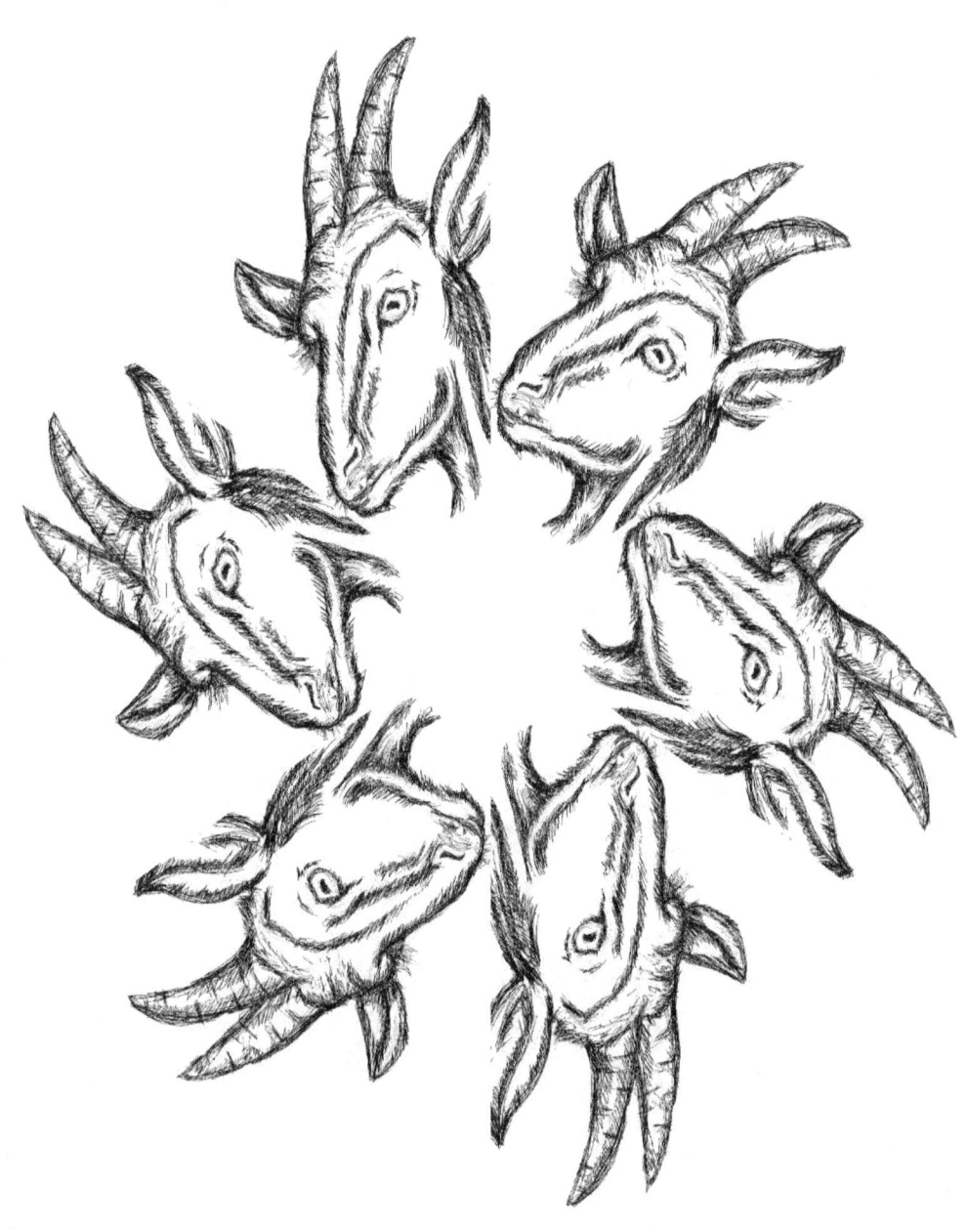

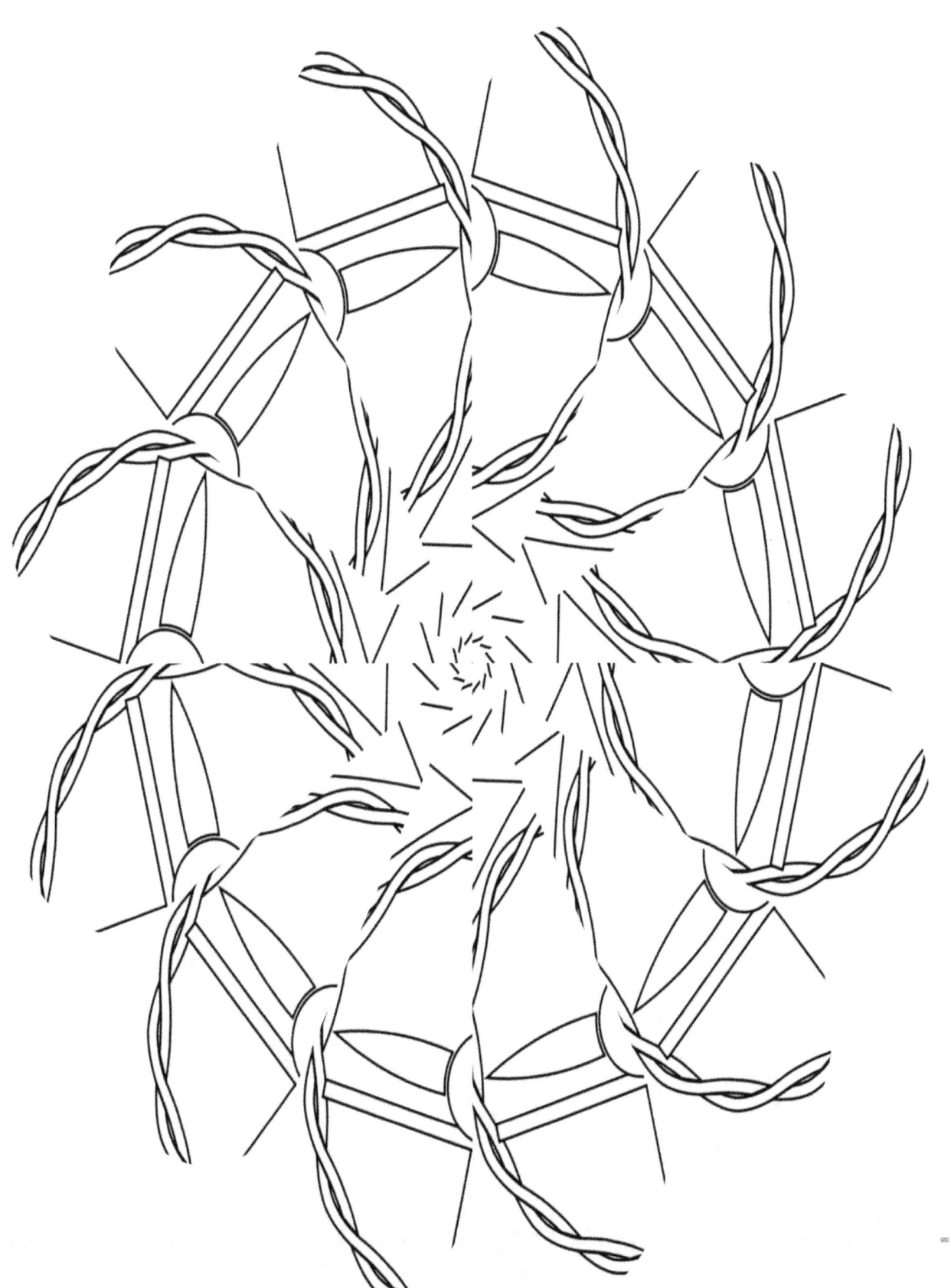

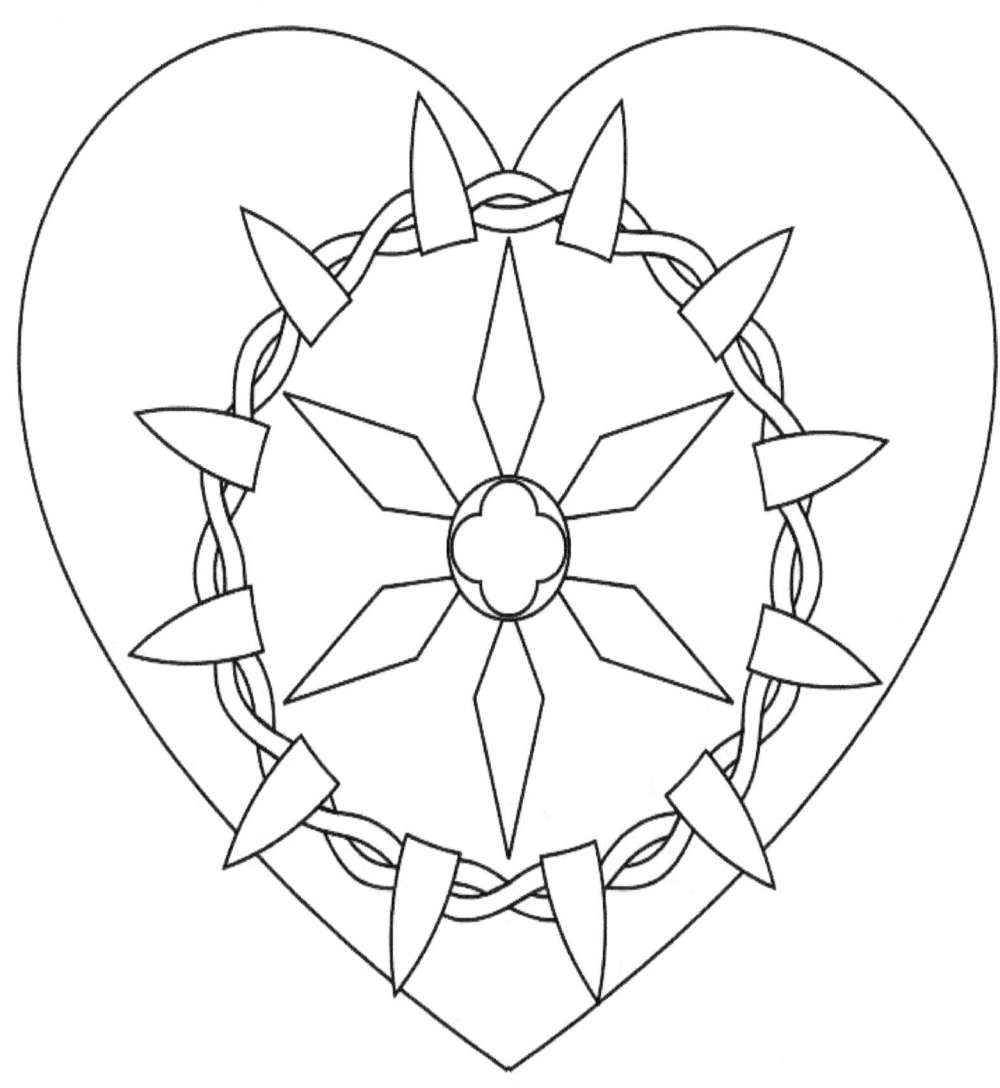

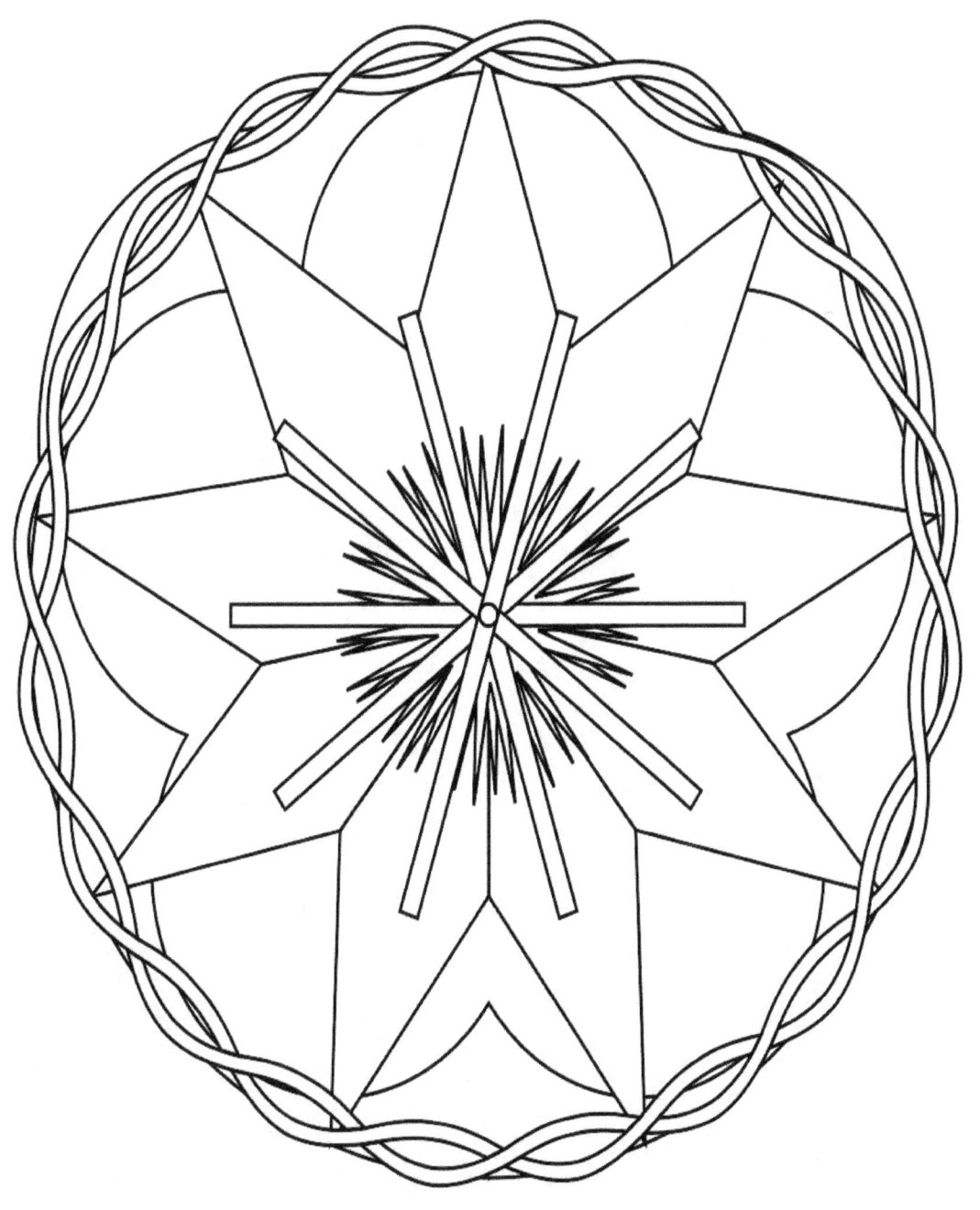

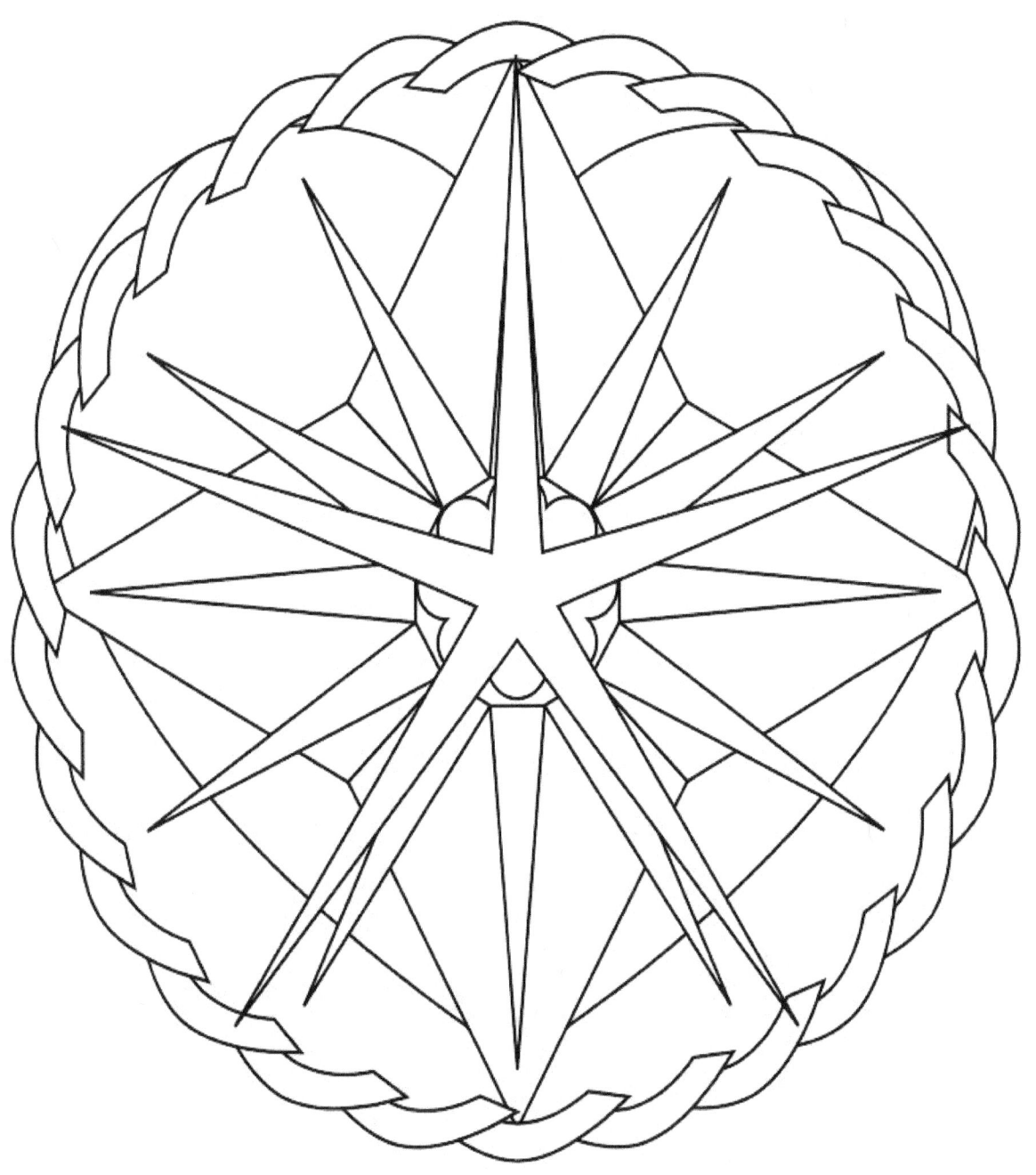

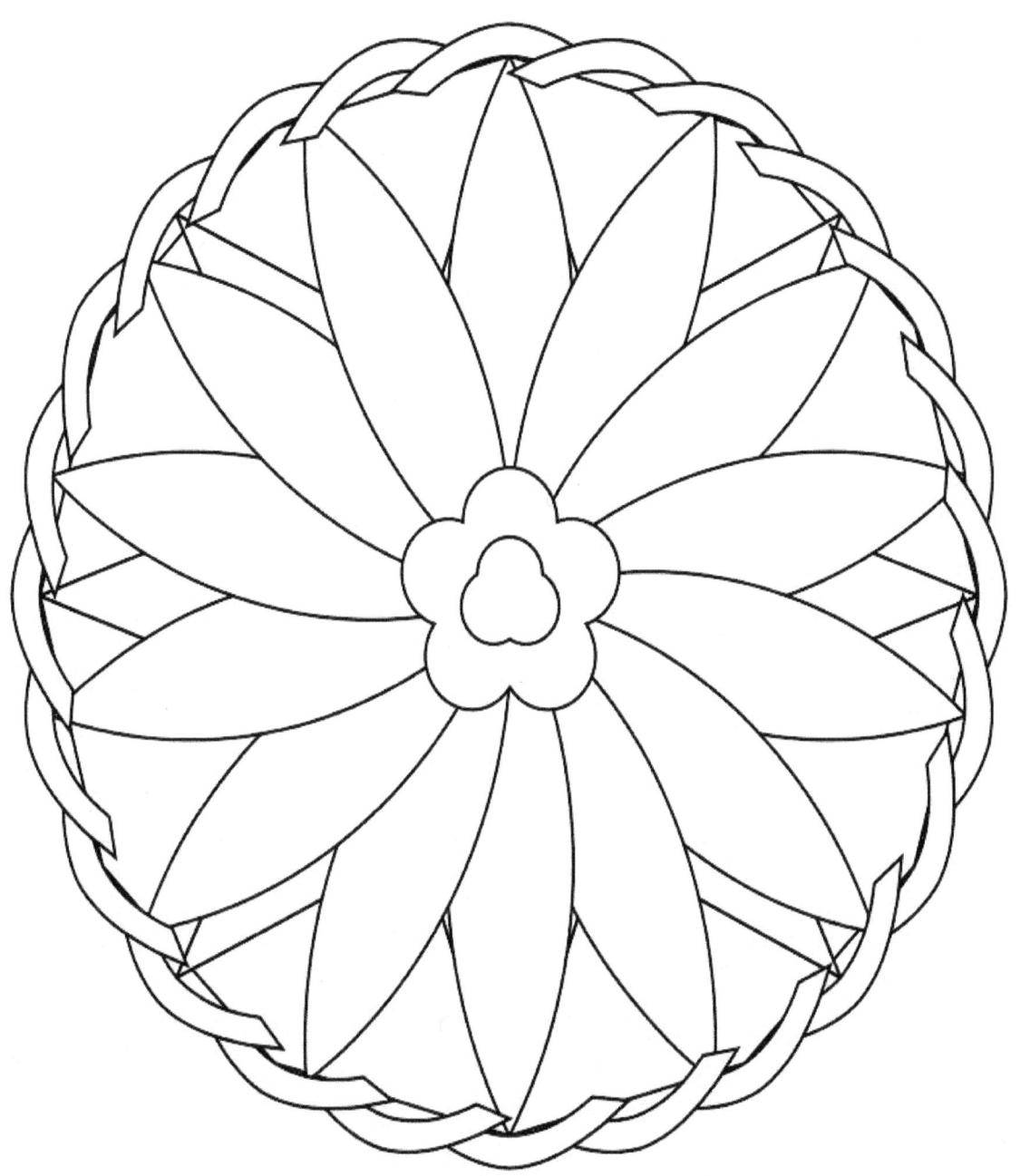

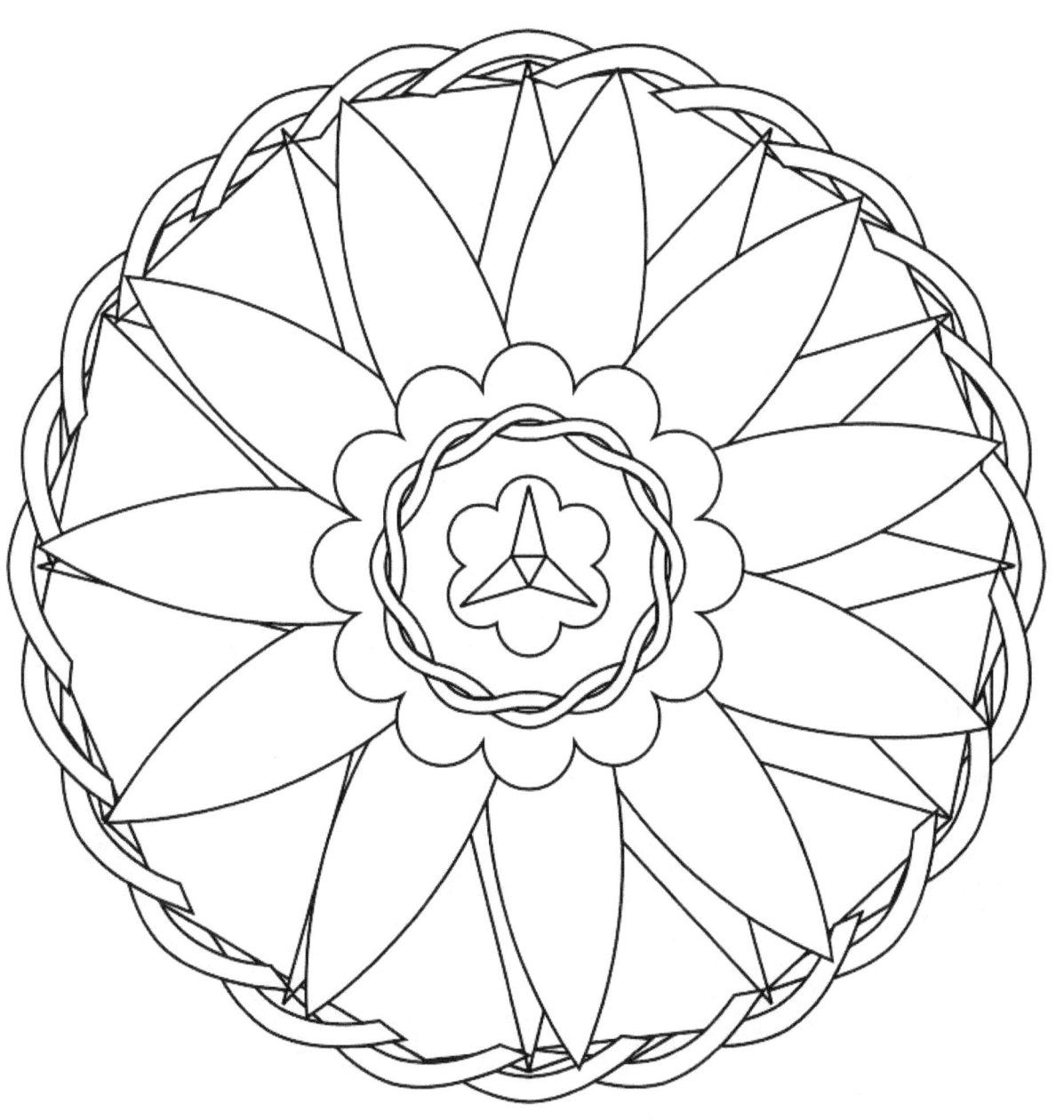

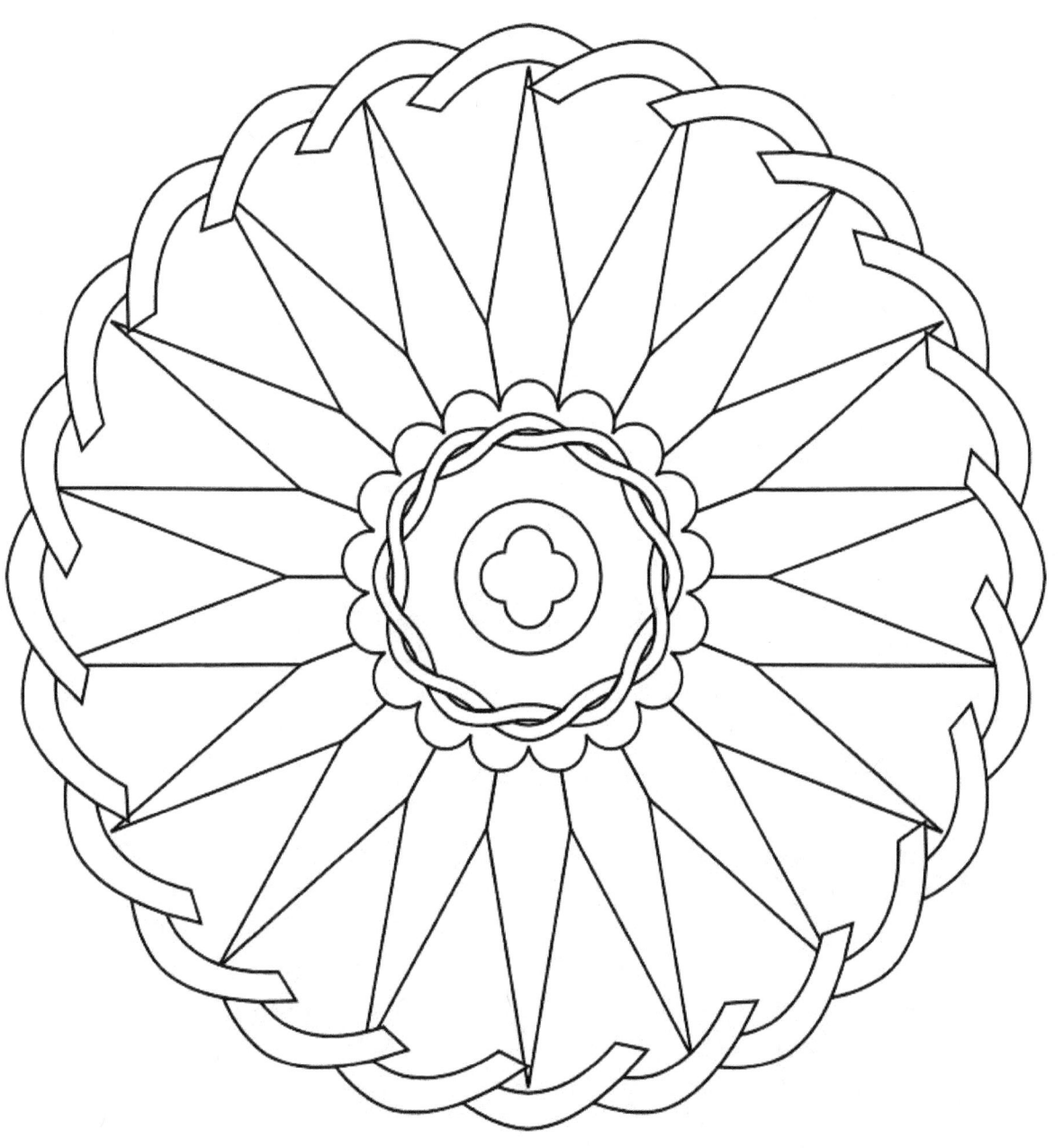

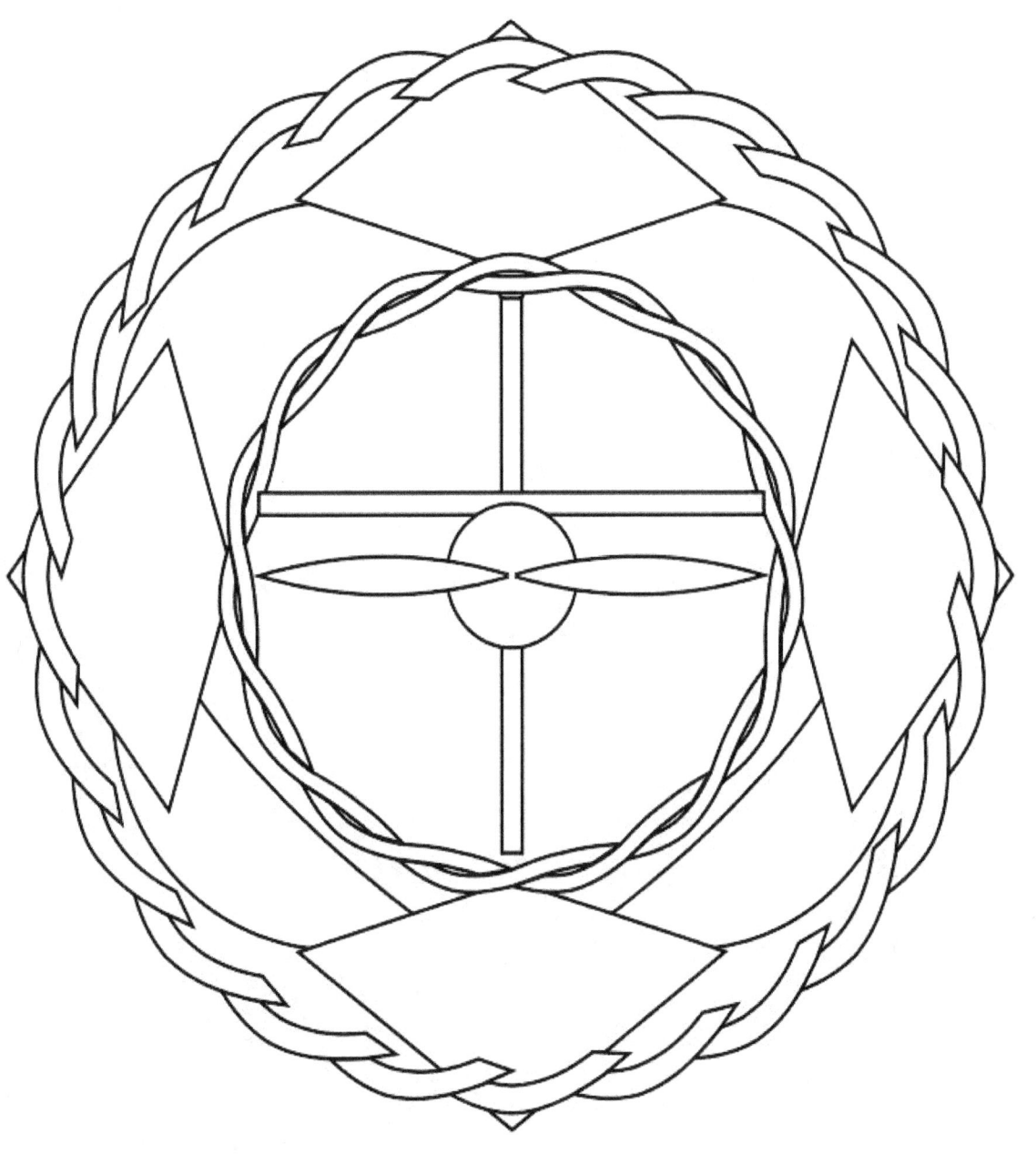

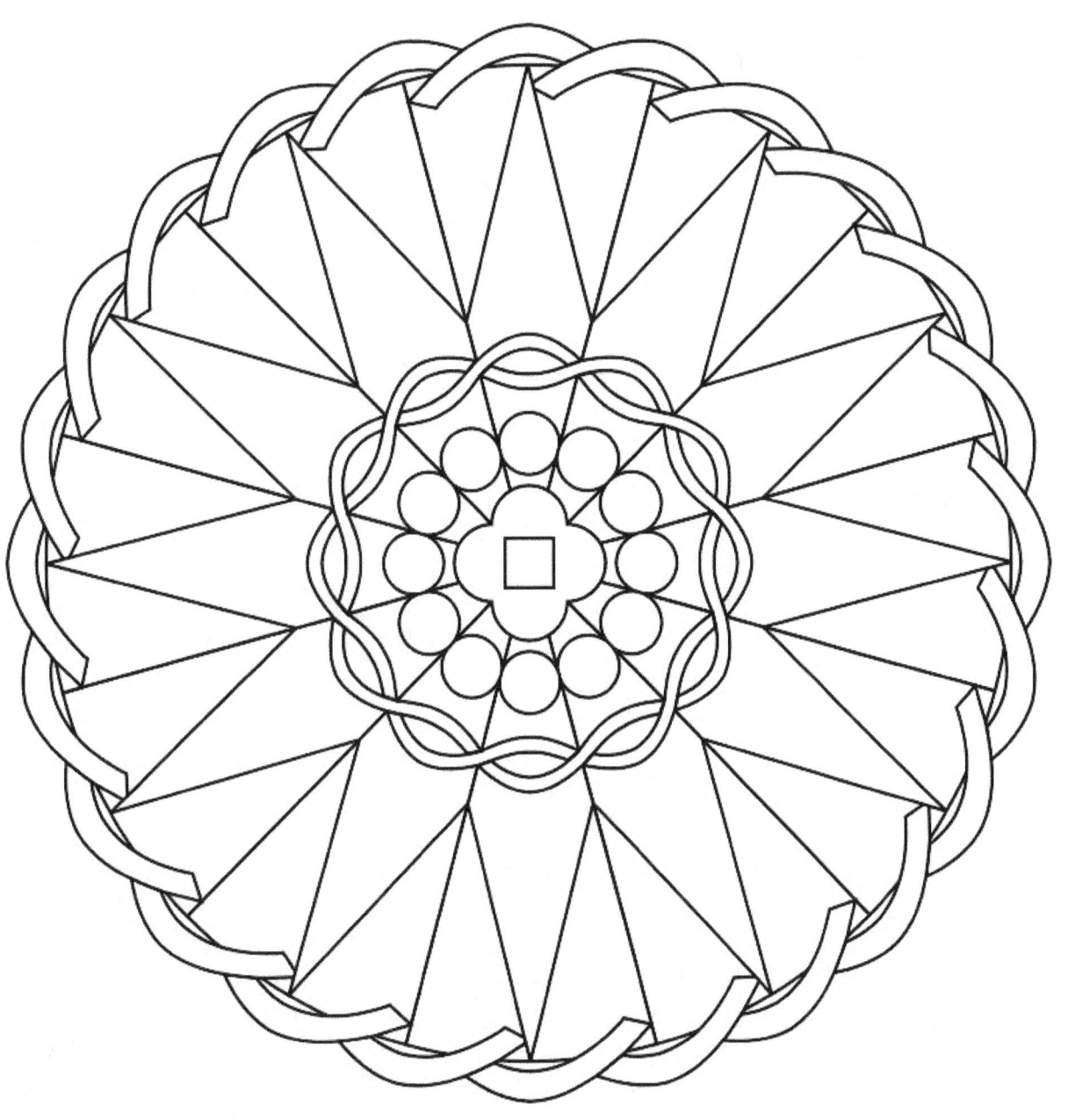

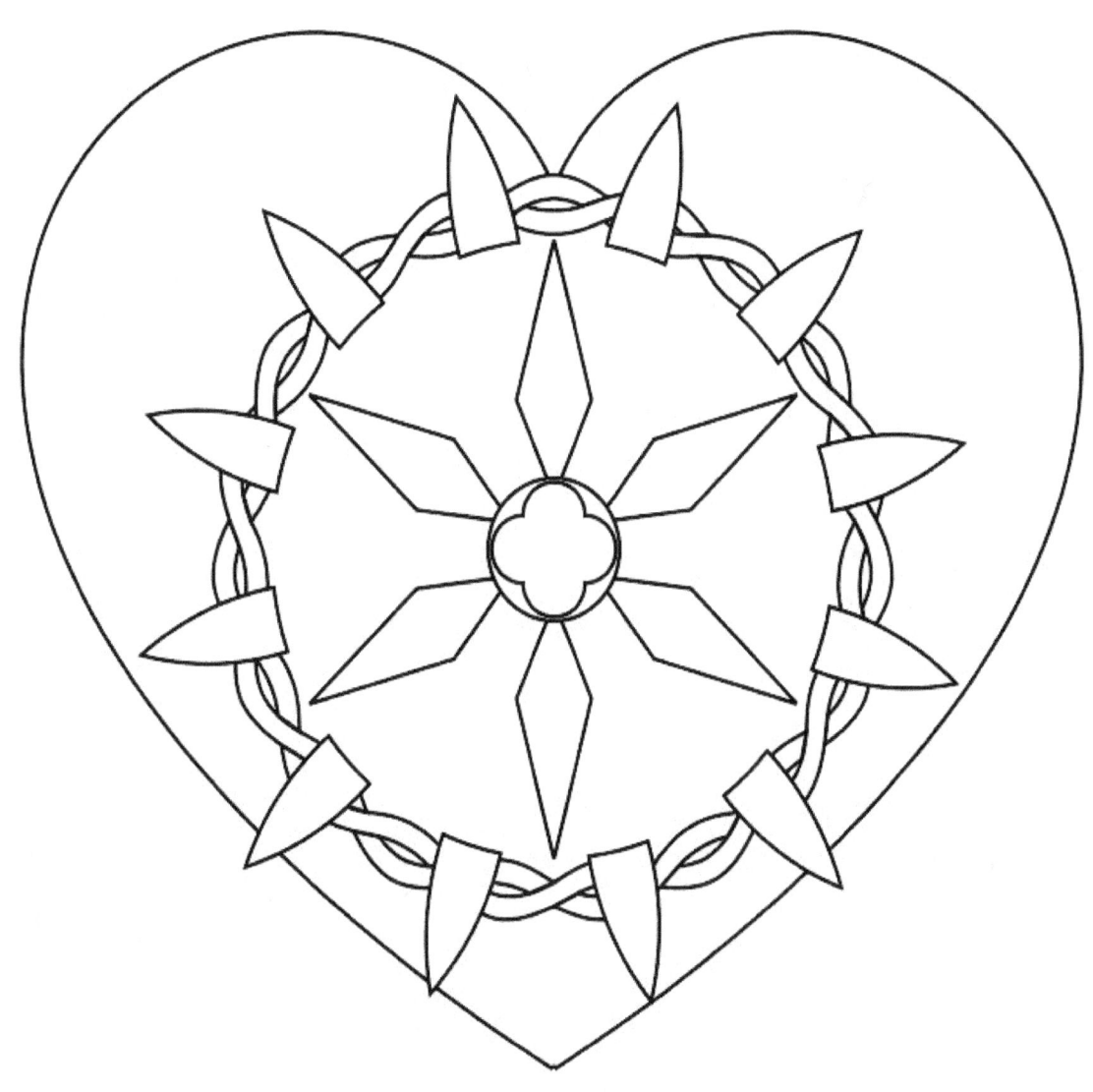

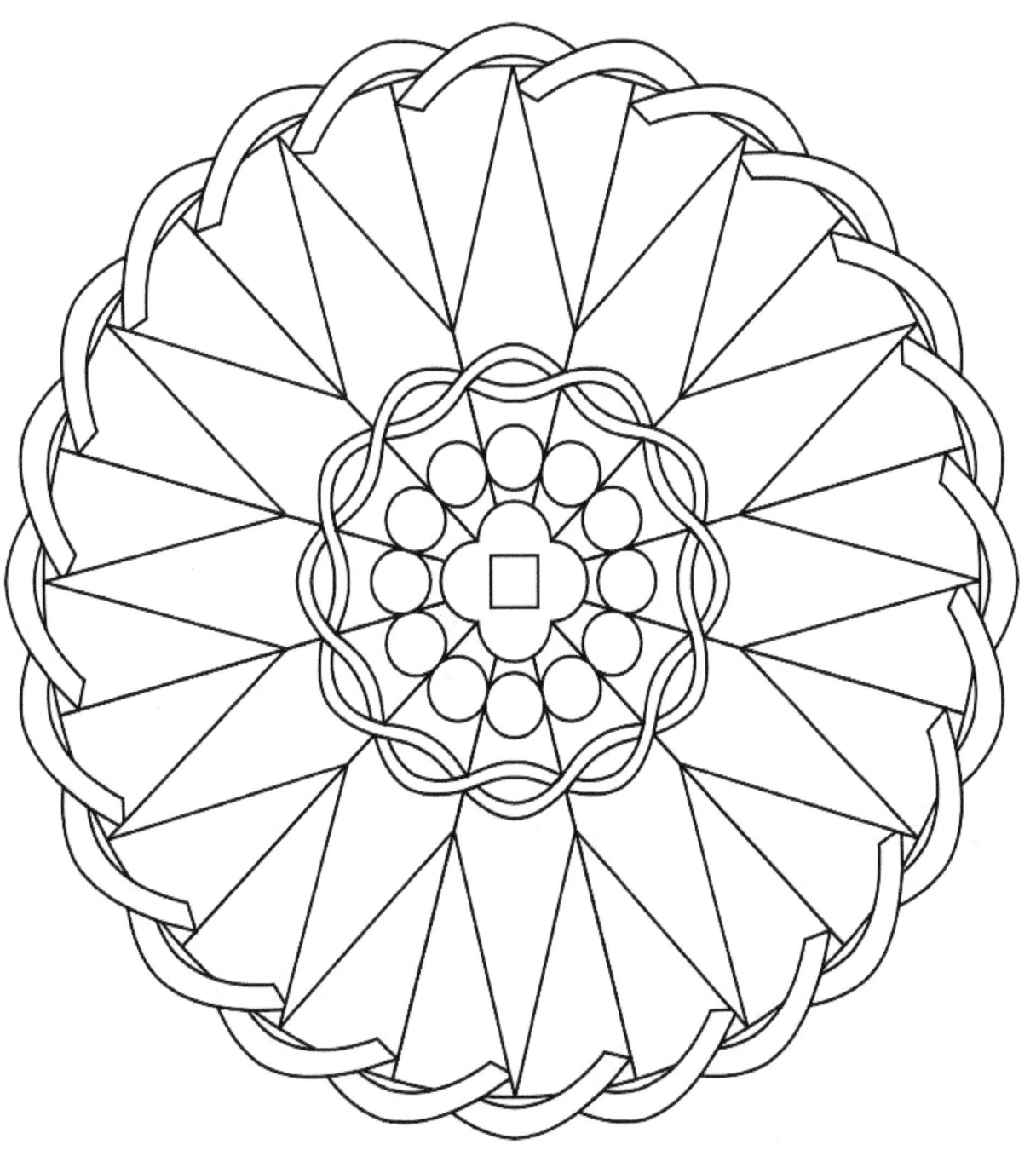

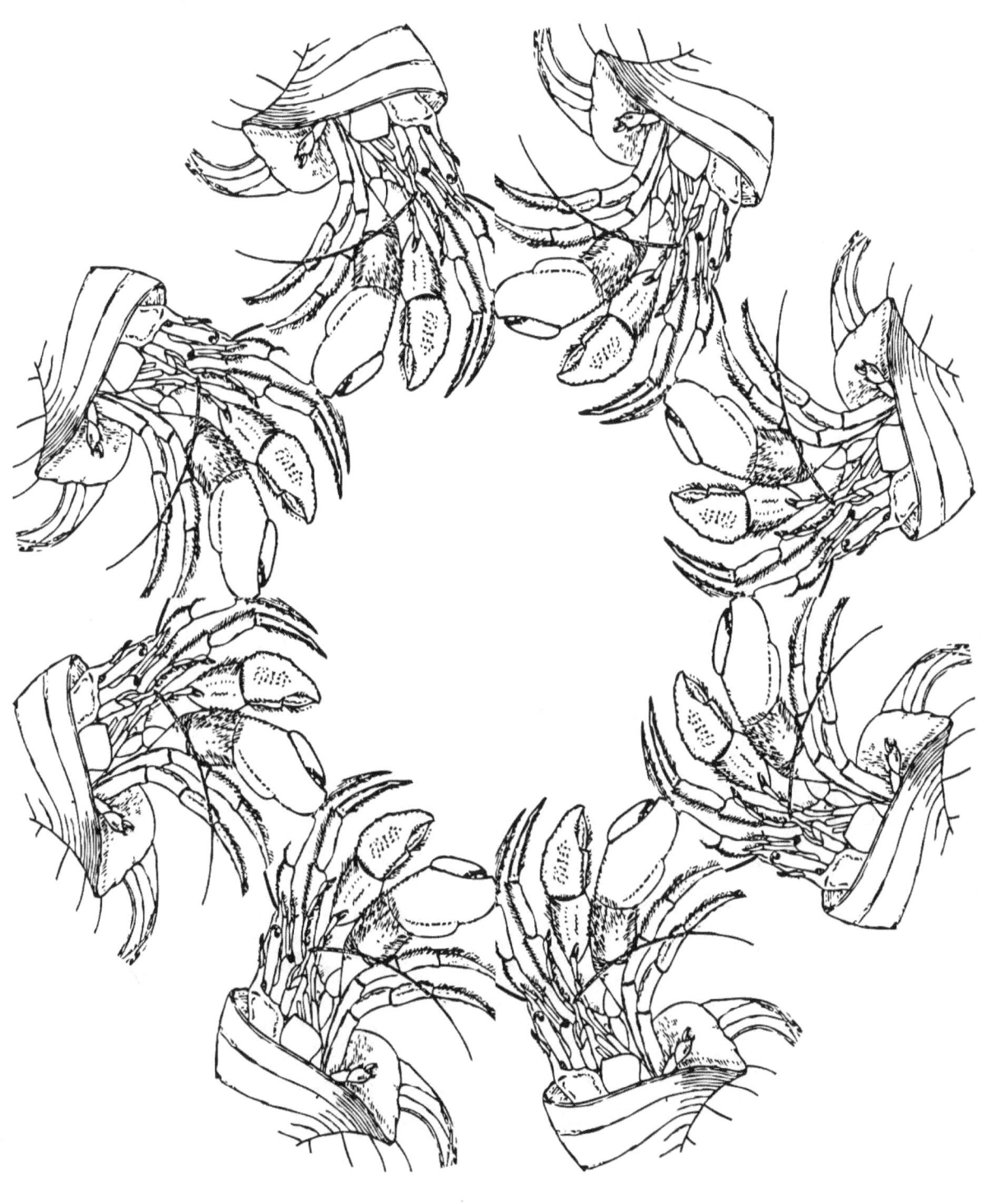

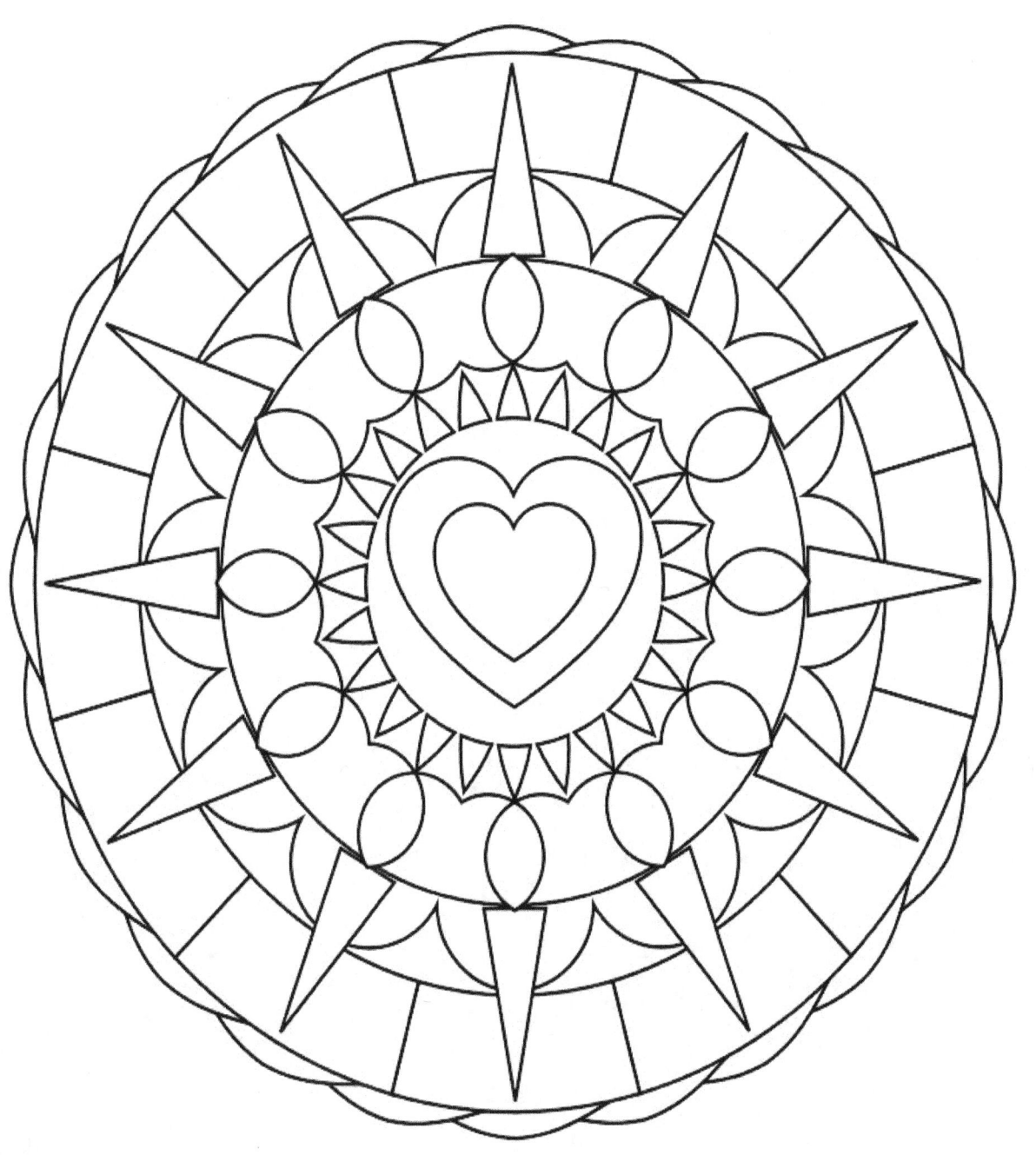

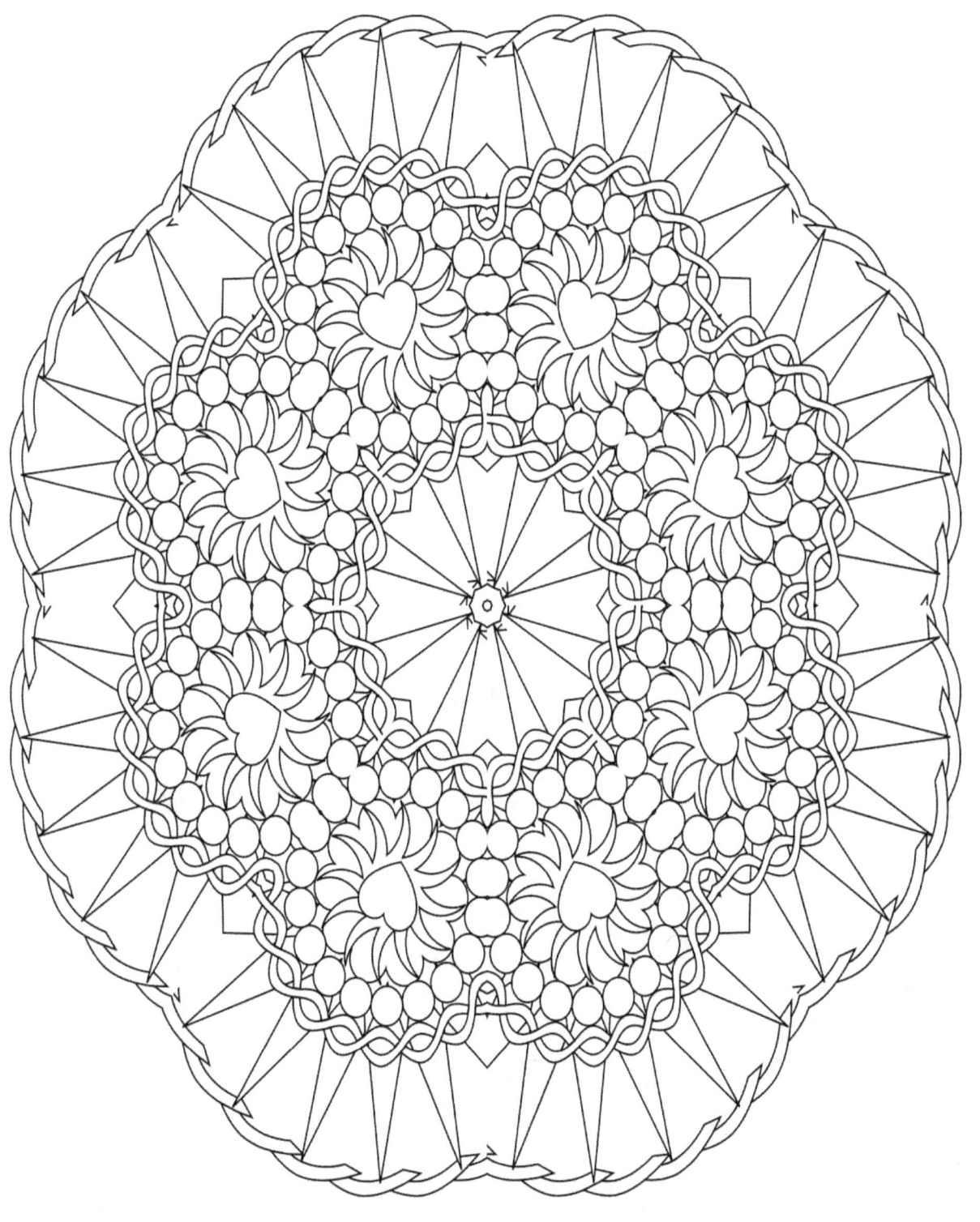

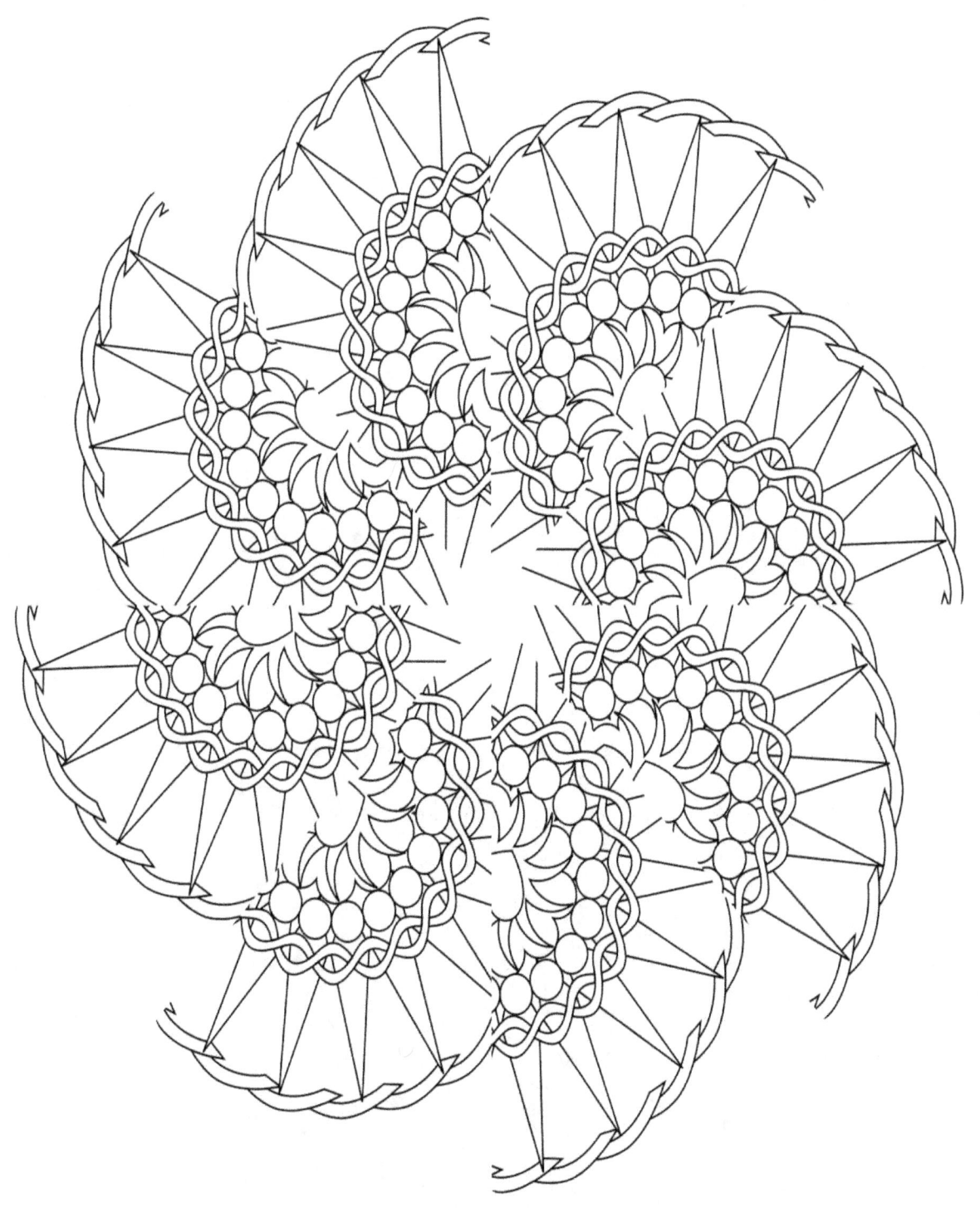

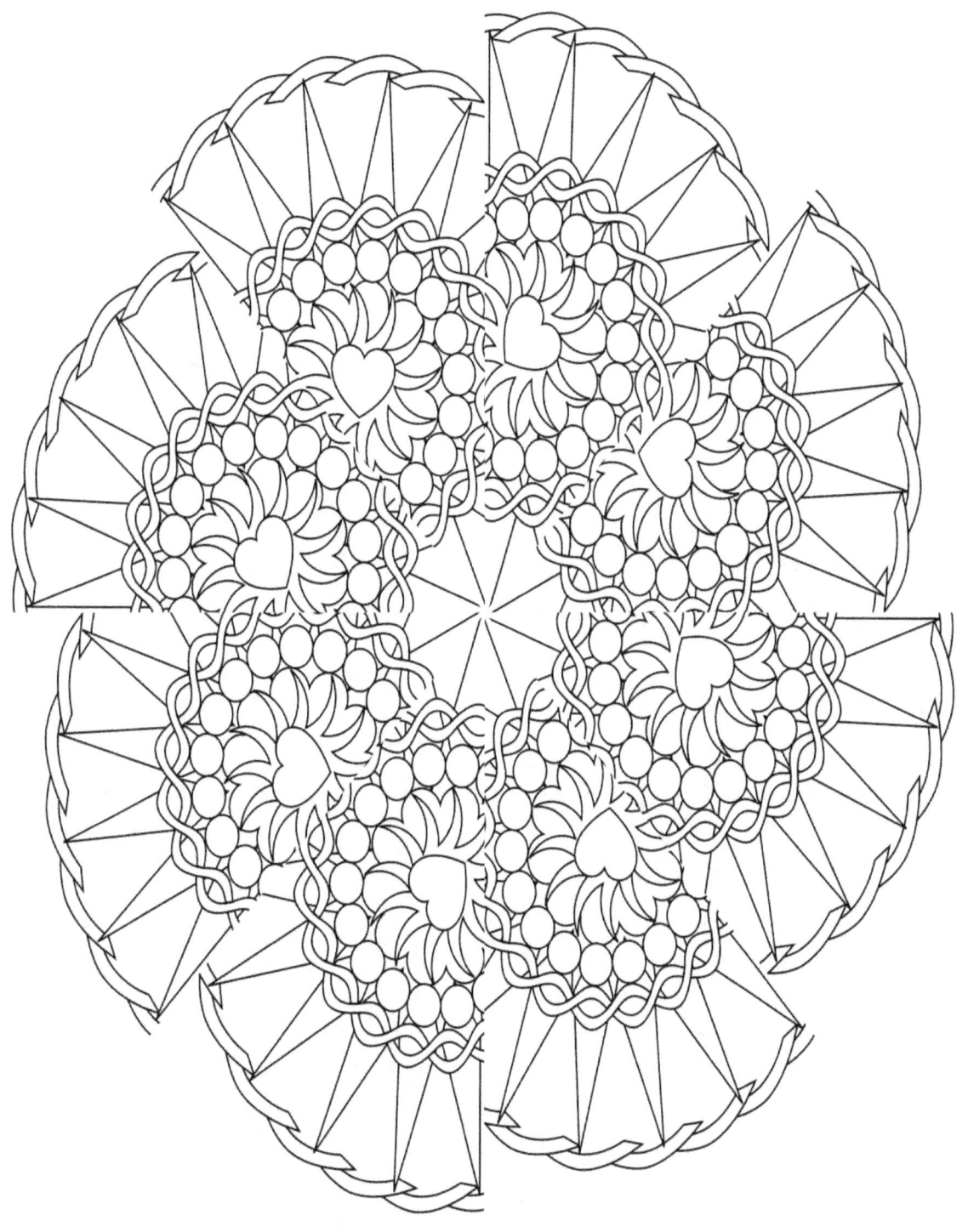

103

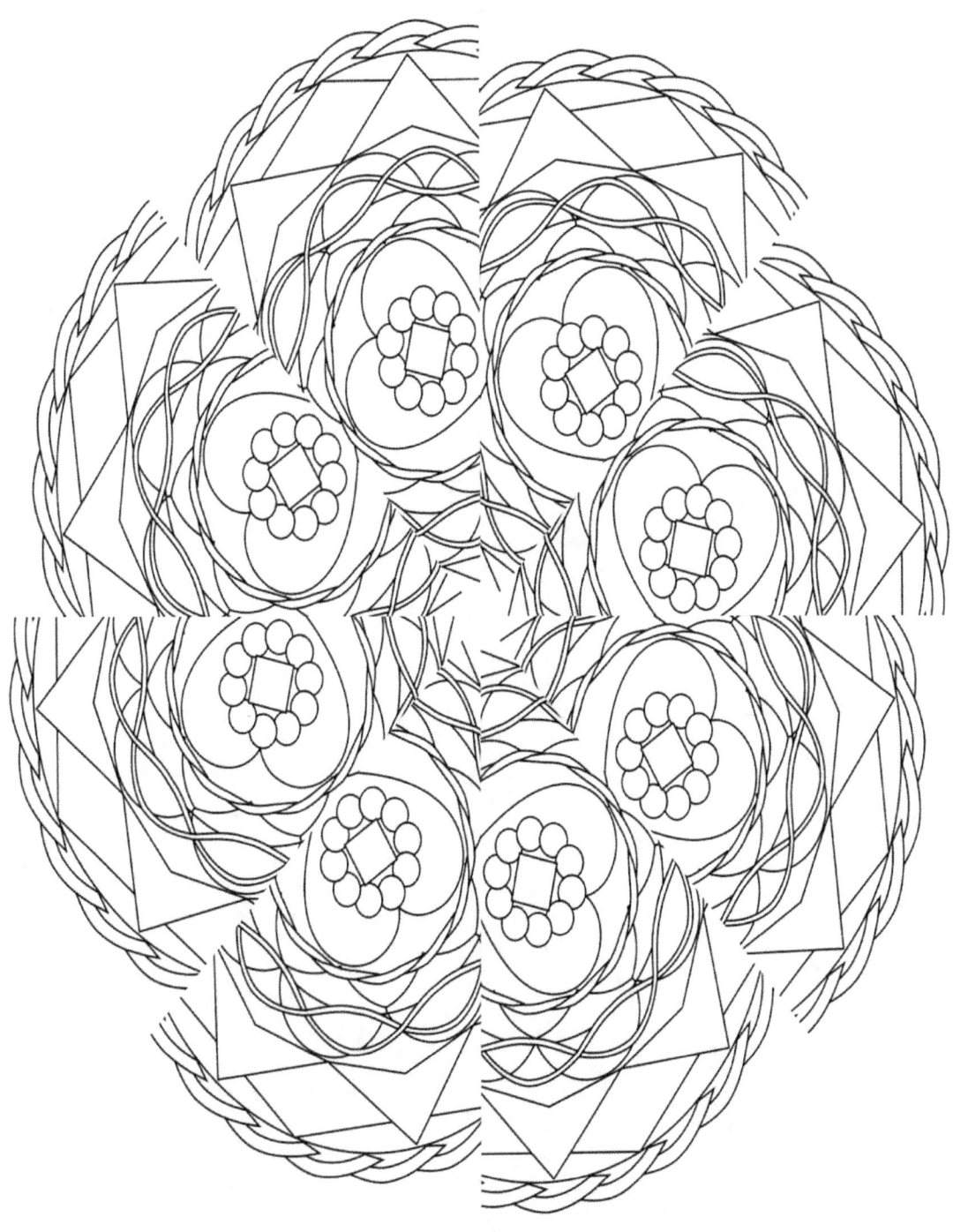

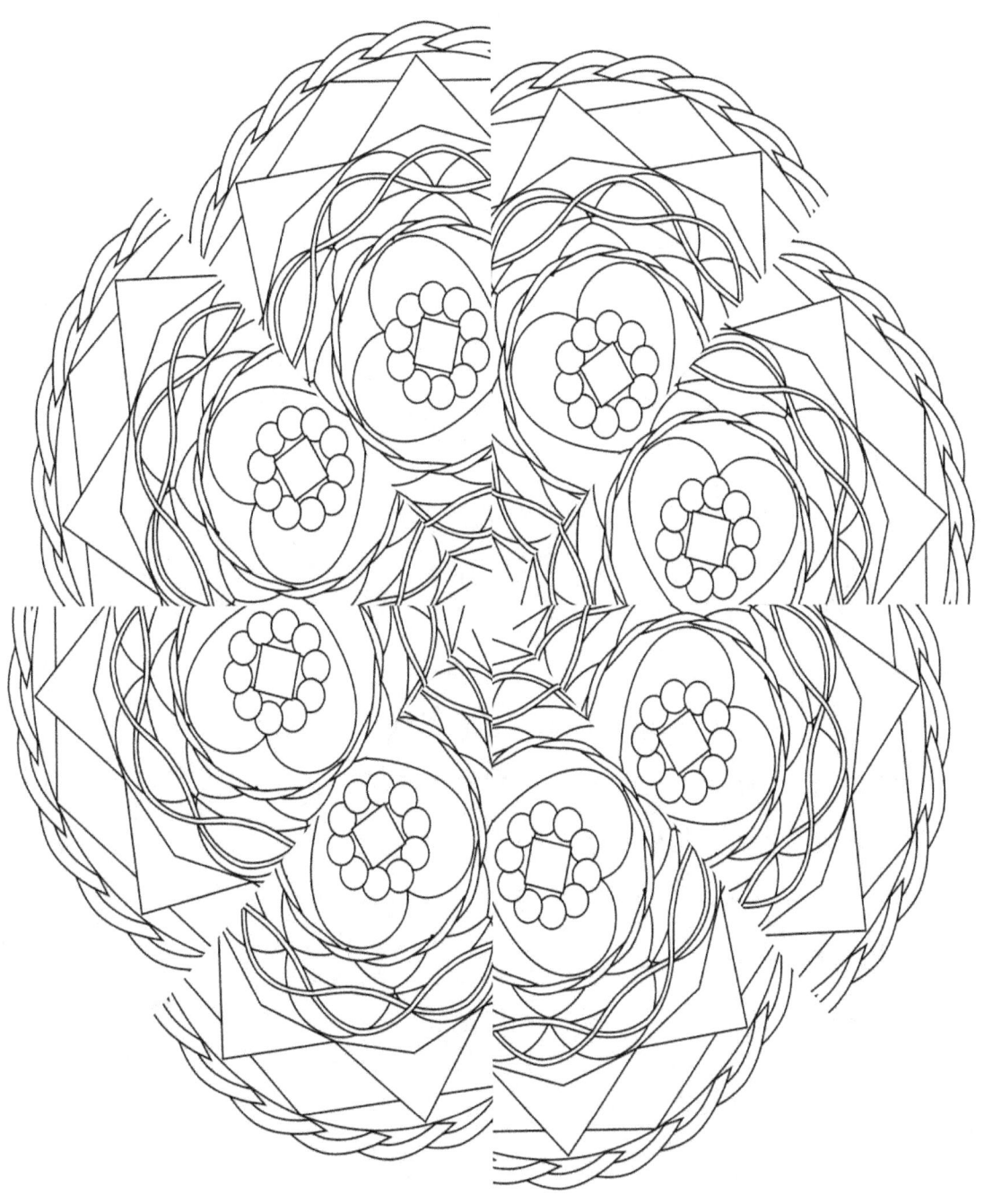

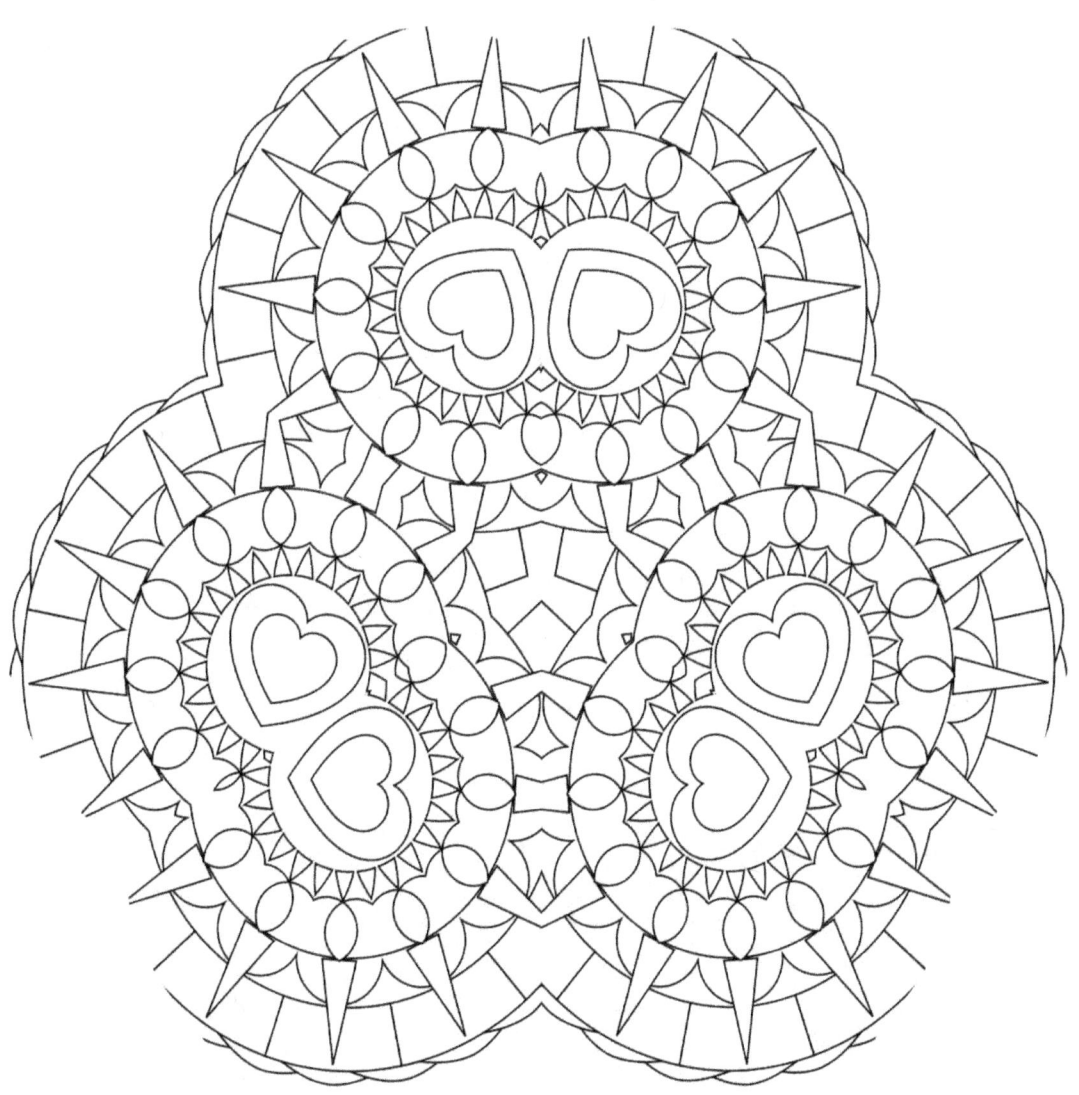

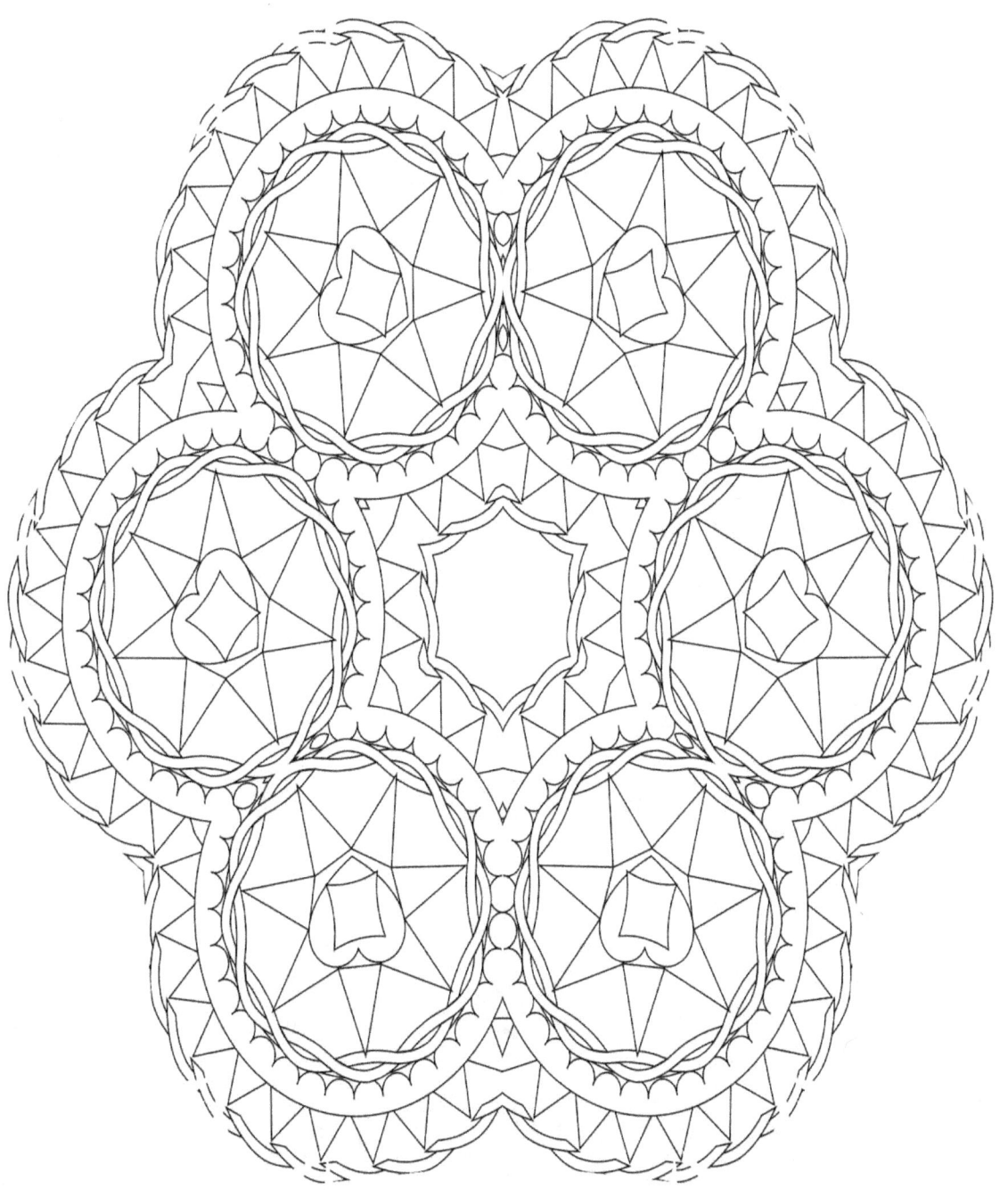

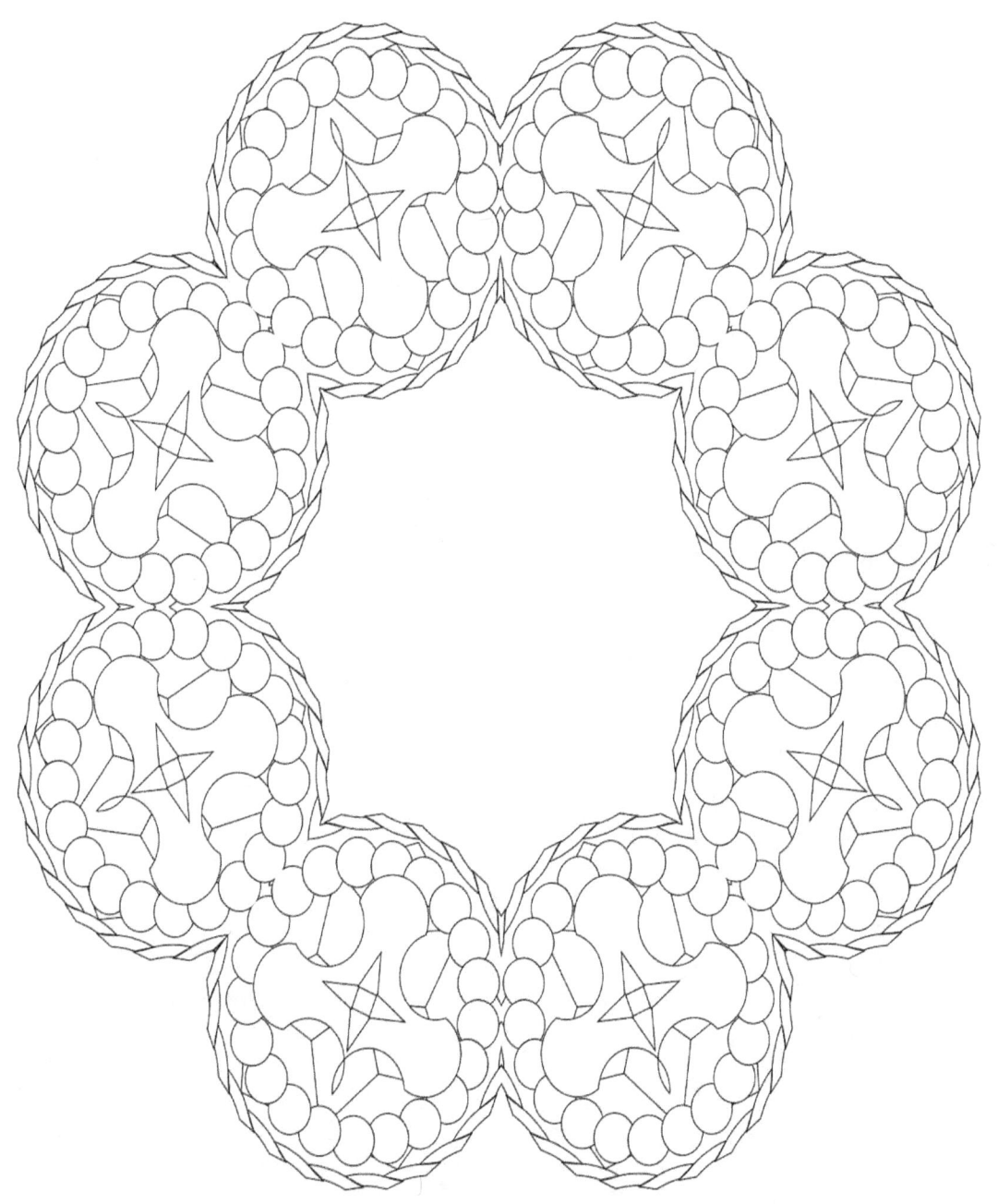

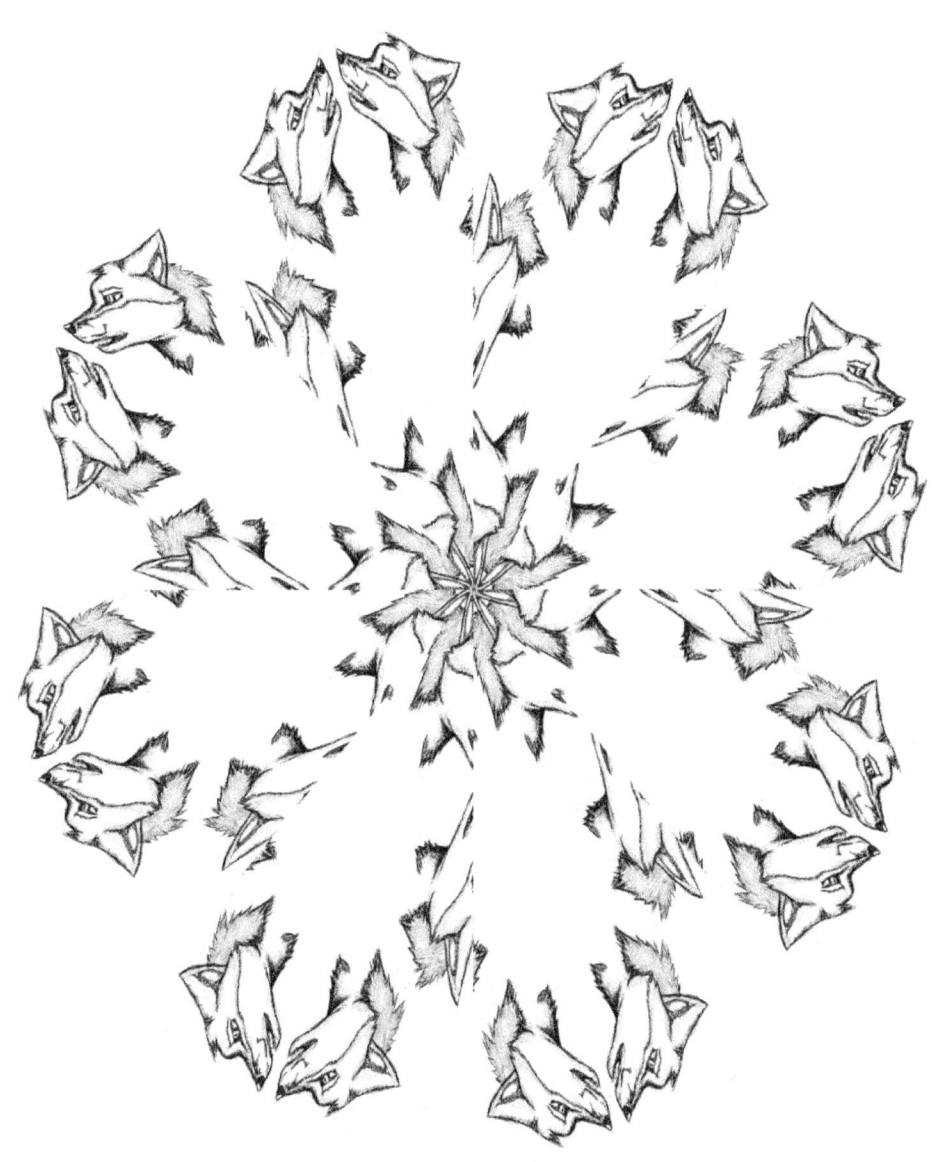

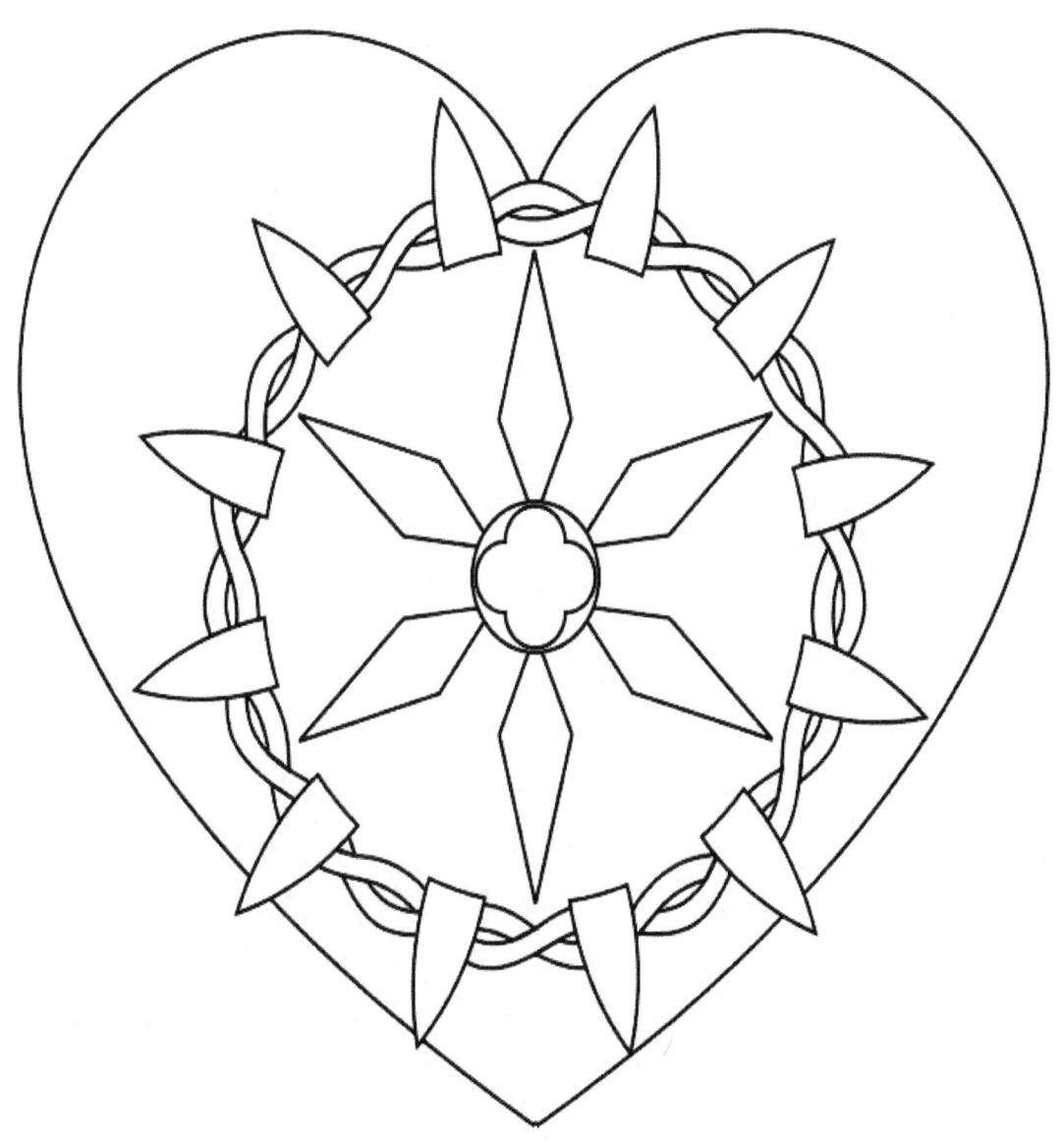

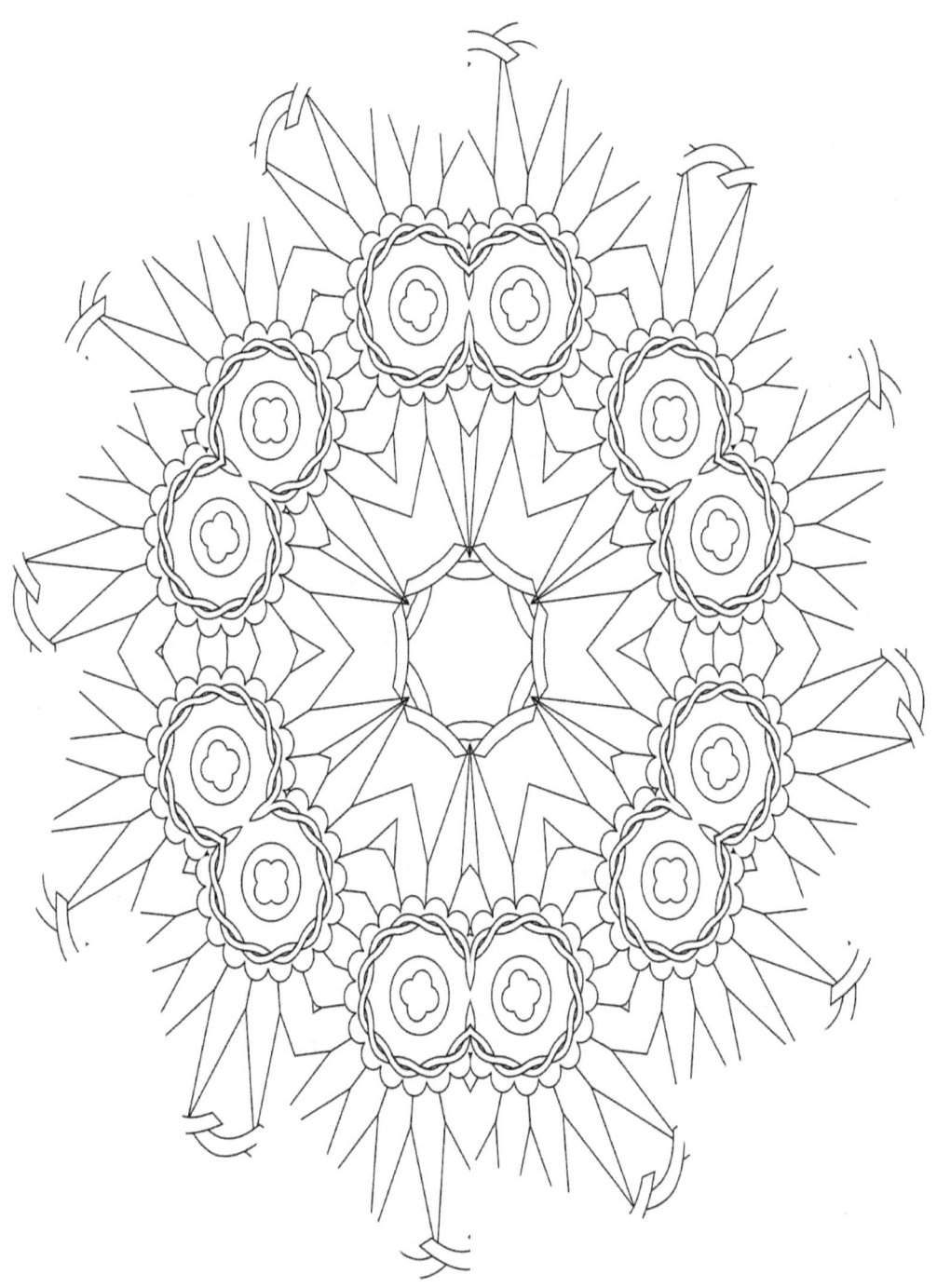

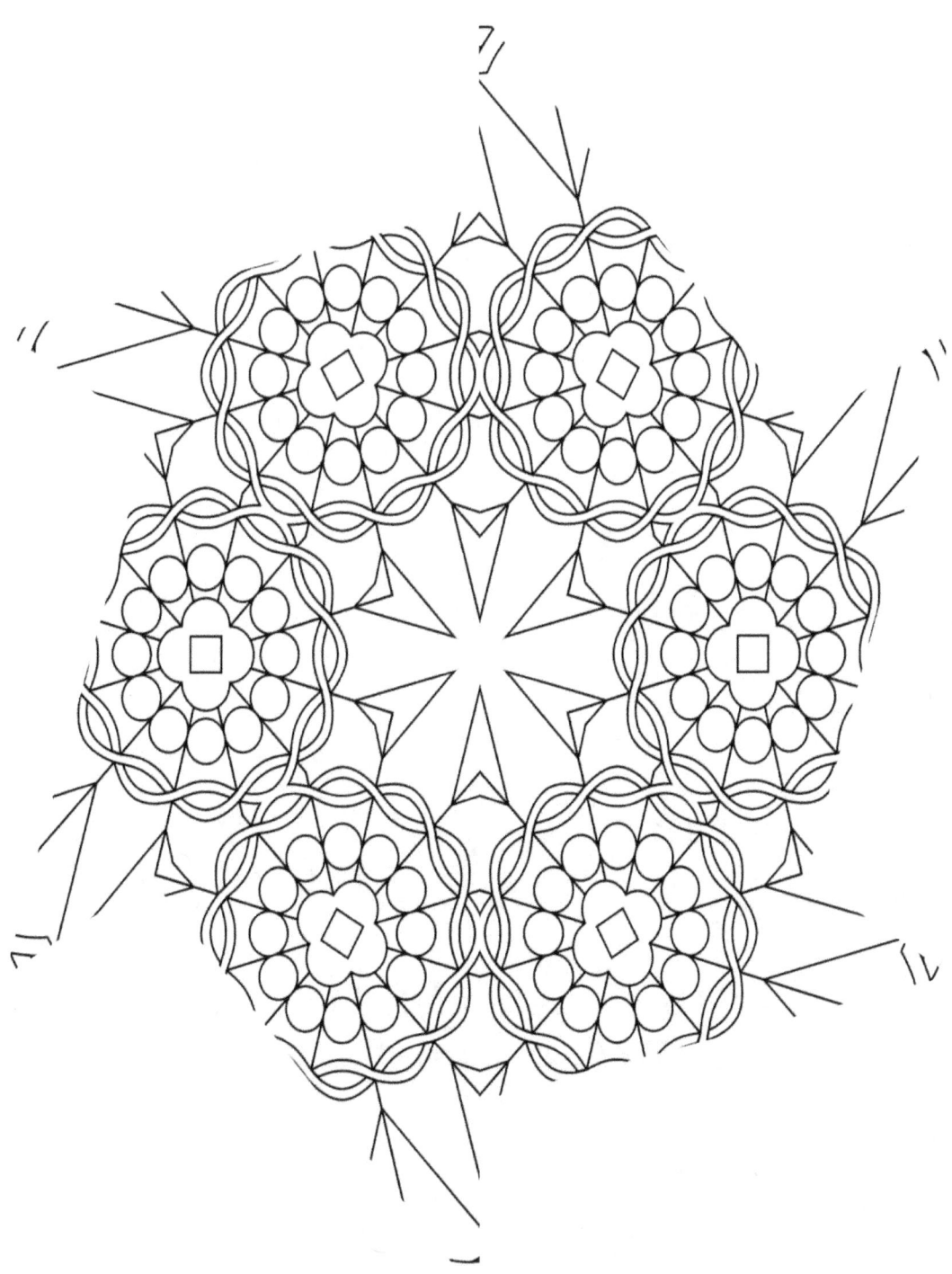

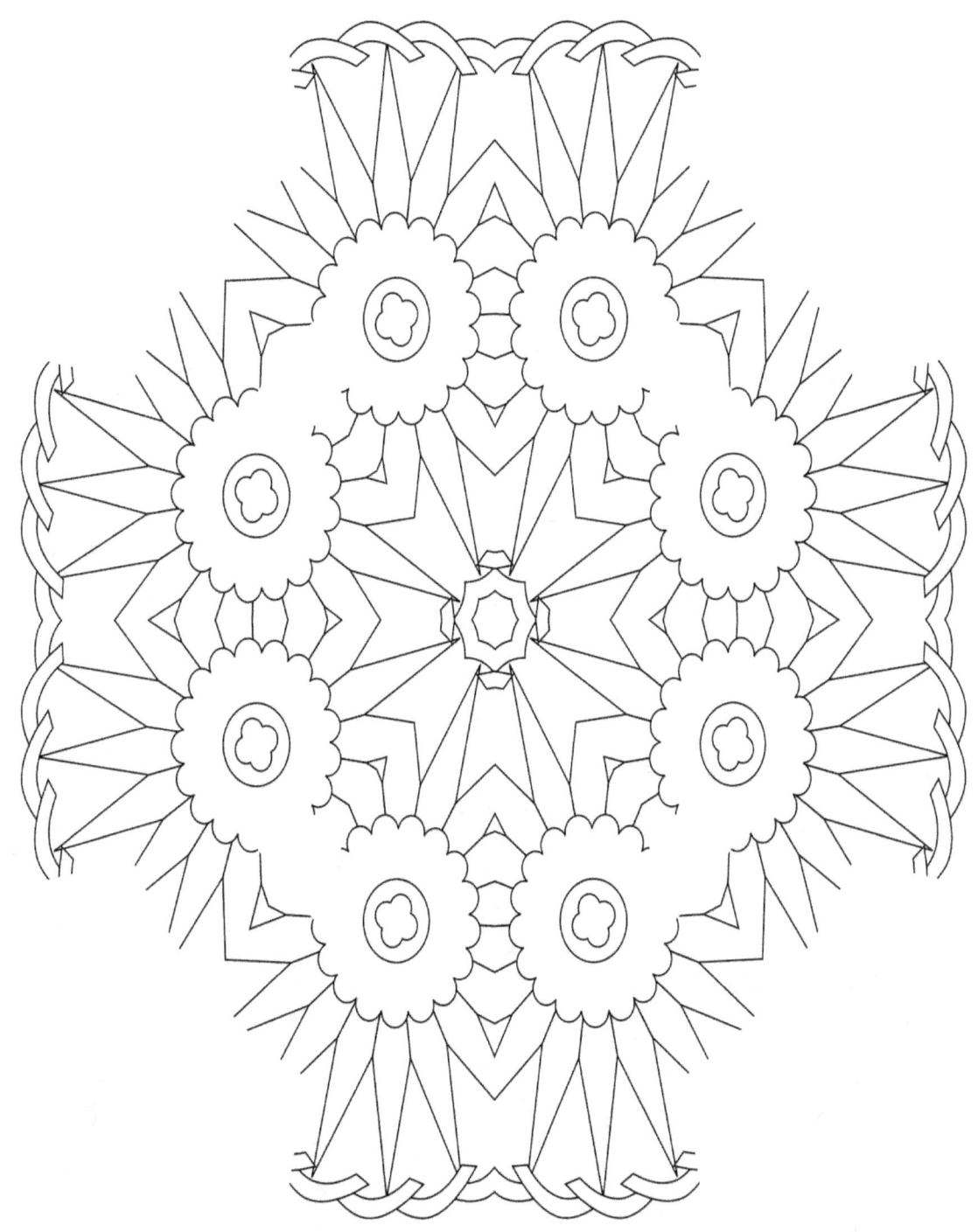

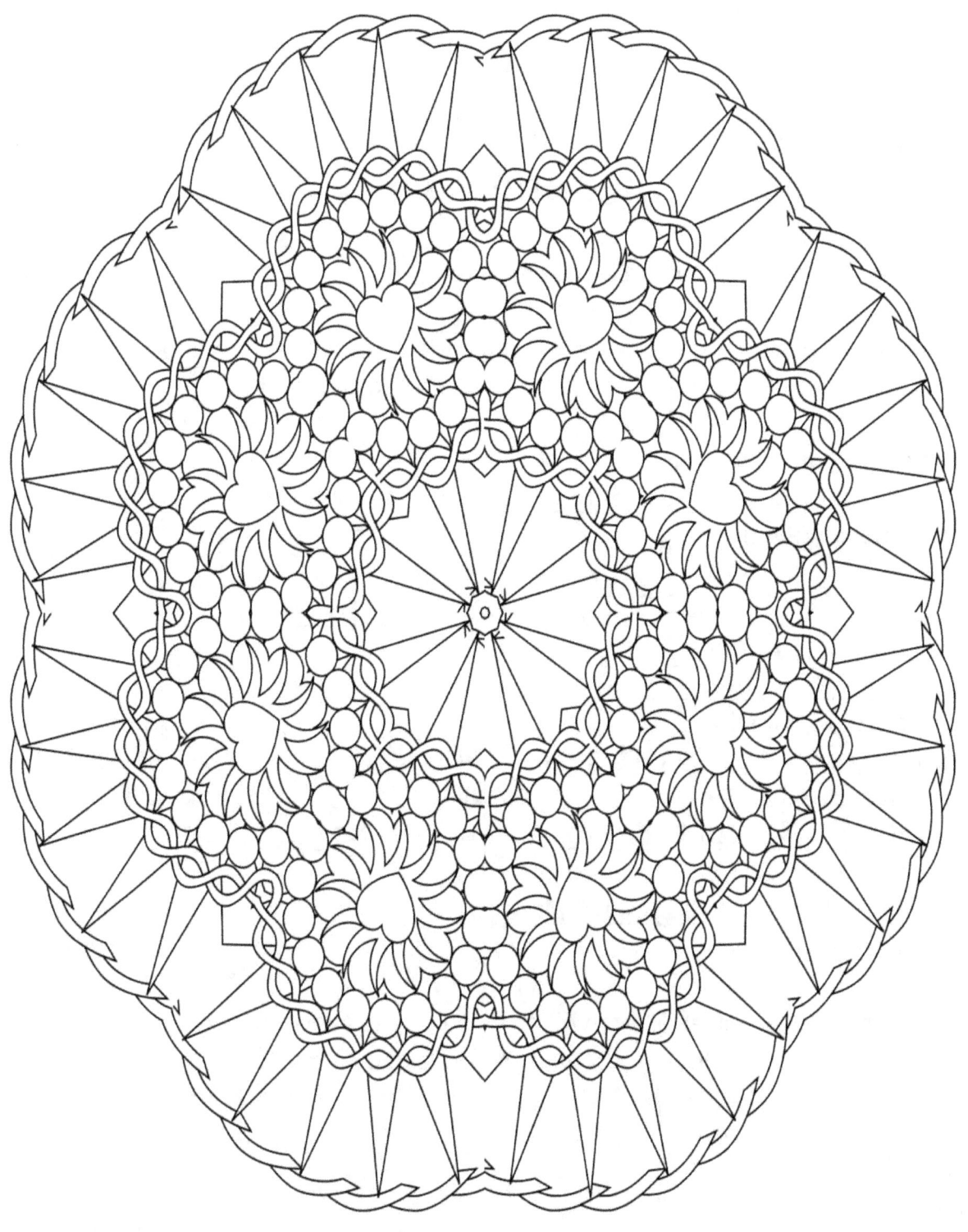

RESOURCE PAGE

The following are some resource you might enjoy.

Buds Free books   http://www.budsfreebooks.com/ This site has a lot of good reading on it. Some are free. some are cheap and some are not.

Other books you might enjoy.

99 Cents Save $100 a year on Laundry Soap

http://amzn.to/PPFpvg

HOW TO GROW YOUR OWN GARDEN BEDDING PLANTS-For Fun And Profit!

http://amzn.to/Q8X7v8

OLD ROVER MY BEST FRIEND

http://amzn.to/XyUvbX

RAISED BED INTENSIVE GARDEN: HOW TO BUILD ONE FOR SELF SUFFICIENCY

http://amzn.to/Tw2jGC

VEGETABLE GARDENING FOR FOOD PRODUCTION AND SELF SUFFICIENCY

http://amzn.to/Tw2LEM

DUMMIES GUIDE TO A 300,000 MILE CAR

http://amzn.to/SQV8HS

Sign up for our newsletter. There will be free images every so often and we will be coming out with a couple of new coloring books each month.

www.ingramcontent.com/pod-product-compliance
Lightning Source LLC
Chambersburg PA
CBHW080415290526
45791CB00008BA/2288